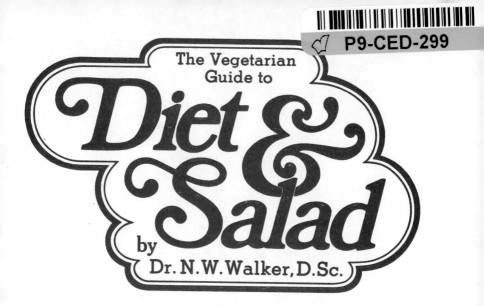

The Vegetarian
Guide to

Diet & Salad

by
Dr. N.W. Walker, D.Sc.

for use in connection with
VEGETABLE and FRUIT JUICES

◆

N.W. WALKER, D. Sc.

Author of:

FRESH VEGETABLE & FRUIT JUICES, What's Missing in Your Body!
VIBRANT HEALTH, The Possible Dream
WATER CAN UNDERMINE YOUR HEALTH
BECOME YOUNGER
BACK TO THE LAND FOR SELF-PRESERVATION
COLON HEALTH – The Key to Vibrant Life
WEIGHT CONTROL – Natural Way To
ENDOCRINE GLANDS CHART
FOOT RELAXATION CHART
COLON THERAPY CHART

NORWALK PRESS
107 N. CORTEZ - SUITE 200
PRESCOTT, ARIZONA 86301
(602) 445-5567

I

THIS BOOK, and many more, including Dr. Walker's other publications, ARE AVAILABLE AT YOUR LOCAL HEALTH FOOD STORE — Your Headquarters for Nutritional Information and Products.

See pages at the back of this Book

for MAIL-ORDER INSTRUCTIONS

Printed in the U.S.A.

CONTENTS

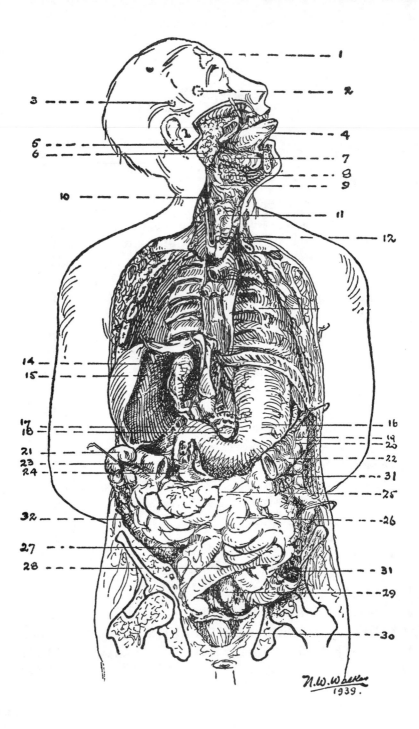

1

2

3

4

5
6

7

8
9

10

11

12

14

15

17
18

16

19
20

21

22

23

24

31

25

32

26

27

28

31

29

30

N.W.Walker
1939.

It is my opinion that the most important subject missing in elementary schools, is ANATOMY.

This sketch is included here to serve as a guide and handy reference.

The numbers indicate the location of the various parts.

1. The Frontal Sinus, in the forehead, above the eyes, where mucus accumulates eventually when we eat excessive amounts of concentrated starches, and drink too much milk.

2. The Pituitary Gland (or Body) is located directly behind and just a little below the level of the bridge of the nose.

3. The Pineal Gland—located in the mid-brain, back, and slightly higher than the Pituitary.

4. The Tongue—one of the most mischievous organs of the human body.

5. The Medulla Oblongata, the central Nerve-telephone-exchange, is situated in the lower middle part of the head, between the upper lip and the base of the skull, just above the Atlas or first cervical vertebra.

6. The Parotid Gland, which becomes swollen and causes Mumps, especially when children and adolescents indulge in excesses of starches and candies.

7. The Sub-Lingual Gland.

8. Sub-Maxillary Gland.

9. The Epiglottis.

10. The Pharynx.

11. The Thyroid Gland, one of the most vital and important glands of the body. It requires Iodine-foods for proper functioning. When improperly nourished causes Goiter.

12. The Larynx.

13. The Spleen is located towards the back of number 19. Back of the Ribs at this point are the Lungs; back of the Lungs, the Stomach, the Splenic Flexure of the Colon, the Spleen, the tip of the Pancreas and the left Kidney.

14. The Gall Bladder—That most essential, though greatly abused gland. The Liver (No. 15) has been raised in this picture, with a hook, to show its location. Its duct leads into the Duodenum (No. 24) to lubricate the intestines with the bile. To remove a Gall Bladder (instead of cleansing the system naturally) deprives the unlucky individual of Nature's means for lubricating the intestines sufficiently.

15. The Liver—The most marvelous laboratory in Creation. Created by Nature to withstand on an average about 40 to 50 years of abuse after birth before perceptible and usually uncomfortable disintegration begins.

16. The Stomach—That organ which controls the Individual, unless the Individual learns to control it.

17. The Pyloric Valve, between the Stomach and Duodenum.

18. The Pancreas—The gland which enables the body to utilize natural sugars (such as are found in raw fruits and vegetables) and which breaks down when refined sugars and starches are used to excess, causing diabetes.

19. The Splenic Flexure of the Colon, or the bend in the Colon leading from the Transverse Colon (No. 22 and No. 23) to the Descending Colon (No. 31).

20. The general location (further back) of the Kidneys.

21. The Hepatic Flexure of the Colon, leading from the Ascending Colon (No. 32) to the Transverse Colon (Nos. 23-22).

22. ⎫ The Transverse Colon, frequently becomes a gas storage balloon
23. ⎭ when tense nerves or impactions of waste matter in the Flexures (Nos. 21-19) prevent the gas from expanding and being expelled. As

a result of improper nourishment this section of the Colon easily loses its tone and then sags, causing what is more picturesquely described as a prolapsus.

24. The Duodenum, or Second Stomach, where the alkaline digestive processes are so frequently interfered with by the presence of acid or acid-forming foods with concentrated starches and sugars, often resulting in ulcerous conditions which individuals enjoy calling their Duodenal Ulcers.

25. The area of the Solar Plexus.

26. The Small Intestines, about 25 feet of perpetual trouble, sooner or later, for those who insist on eating what they want when they want it.

27. The Appendix, that marvelous safety gland whose secretion prevents gas-forming bacteria and other noxious germs from passing into the Small Intestines from the Colon. Once known as the Society Topic, and also as the professional dividend standby, it has of late been allowed to function more normally since the education of the laity in the use of frequent enemas and skillful colonic irrigations.

28. The Bladder is in this region.

29. The Sigmoid Flexure of the Colon leading from the Descending Colon (No. 31) to the Rectum (No. 30).

30. The Rectum, the cesspool of the body, which should be washed out with enemas or colonic irrigations quite often.

31. The Descending Colon.

32. The Ascending Colon.

THIS BOOK IS DEDICATED,

With infinite love to all who in their hour of darkness, doubt and suffering are seeking a beam of light to guide their steps across the muddy streams of greed, arrogance and educated ignorance, and with affection and infinite compassion, to those whose background and environment precludes their acceptance of the fundamental principles and the laws of Nature, which the Materialist can sometimes sense but not grasp.

Wisdom may only be obtained
through Truth and
Knowledge.

INTRODUCTION

Human nature is all too often obstinate, stubborn and perverse, refusing to be confused by facts, and is traditionally oblivious or heedless to experience, and to plain common sense.

It seems incomprehensible that supposedly intelligent people can become victimized by claims and statements conceived to misinform and to misguide.

Nature has provided man with all the basic means with which to build his body from birth to old age to a state of maximum health, which includes the joy of living with abundant energy, vigor and vitality, and a happy long span of life.

These basic means are few, and they are physically represented in our natural foods, first and foremost.

The secret of achieving an abundant life consists in proper nourishment, coupled with sufficient rest and the control of emotions. Actually, this is no secret at all!

This past century has spawned a vast number of research, manufacturing and marketing organizations whose sole aim is the profit to be derived from a perversion of natural foods cheaply manufactured and sold at the highest price that traffic will bear.

The uninformed gullible public, ignorant of what constitutes basic, natural, correct nutrition, has accepted sales indoctrination and misinformation, and buys its food blindly, utterly unaware of the fact that instead of nourishing the body constructively, such food may actually cause a chain reaction of degenerating processes. This has resulted in our Nation having become the best fed, yet the most undernourished, ailing and sick Nation this world has ever known.

Light, at last, is perhaps beginning to manifest. The Youth of today is searching for a means to overcome this deception. People who have spent a lifetime steeped in the fallacy that drugs, pills and hypodermic injections are cure-alls, people who have habitually, sometimes for years on end, made needless visits to offices in which they had vainly pinned their hopes and faith, so many of these people who never dreamed of arguing the fallacy of their expectations, are today, to their utter surprise and amazement, finding that Nature's simple means to achieve health are the Creator's medicine for what ails us.

7

ORGANIC FOOD & ENZYMES

LIFE! What does man prize above and beyond everything else? HIS L I F E ! Right?

LIFE is one thing that no scientist, chemist, inventor or other kind of human being has ever been able to create.

LIFE is the sole and exclusive creative prerogative of Almighty God, our Creator. However, Almighty God has given to human beings the privilege and prerogative of exercising free will, self will.

Self preservation is the aim of every man, woman and child . . . Or is it?

Even a child can understand that one cannot have life and death at one and the same time. LIFE begets LIFE, and in no other way can LIFE be begat!

This being the case, is it not intelligent, rational, discerning and wise to consider and to conclude that the regeneration and replenishment of the life in your body must essentially come from the LIFE inherent in the food you eat? That the LIFE present in such nutrition has the property and the ability to regenerate and to revitalize the LIFE within the cells and tissues of your body, daily and constantly?

How can one eat LIFE? Natural foods, in their natural raw state contain life in the atoms and molecules composing them. Such atomic LIFE is classified as ENZYMES.

Food which is replete with Enzymes and which has been grown on properly prepared soil, is organic food. Food in which Enzymes have been destroyed by excessive heat is INorganic.

To clarify the definition of ORGANIC and INorganic, we use ORGANIC in referring to food which has been grown from unprocessed seed in soil which is replete with earthworms as a result of proper composting and complete absence of chemical fertilizers and poison sprays.

Of course all raw food is organic, but not all raw food is grown organically!

Organically grown food means more than food grown without sprays and chemical fertilizers. Actually it takes years to build up a depleted or chemically poisoned soil. The present condition of the soil and how it has been used or abused in the past determines the number of years it will take to build it up to a state of NATURAL FERTILITY by the use of compost and good organic farm practice. Only then will the soil be truly fit to be planted with seeds that will grow beautiful and healthy vegetation which repels pests, germs and disease — just as a healthy body repels sickness.

The reason we have today so much sickness and disease is not only due to the present day commercial system of producing such vast volumes of deficient food, but also because our soil is sick from lack of proper care and nourishment.

A healthy soil = healthy food = a healthy body.

As Enzymes form the fundamental basis of nutrition, they should have our first consideration in the choice of our food. Enzymes are not substances which man can create, nor are they capable of being synthesized for use as supplements for constructive purposes.

Enzymes are the life-principle in every live, organic atom and molecule, whether such atoms compose vegetation or are the atoms and molecules in the constitution of the human and animal bodies.

Only Almighty God can create LIFE. Consequently only God can create Enzymes.

The Enzymes in the body give the spark of activity to every cell and tissue, as well as to their functions, so long as the body is alive. The moment the body dies, the life represented by its Enzymes is dissipated, at which time the atoms and molecules and the cells and tissues composing the anatomy are no longer subject to regeneration and begin to decompose.

Enzymes in your food are the life in the atoms and molecules constituting the food.

DO YOU KNOW THAT YOUR BODY HAS A SEWER?

Let us be frank and honest about it: No one man has all the answers. Nevertheless, the very BEST of DIETS can be no better than the VERY WORST, if the sewage system, the eliminative organs in your anatomy, is clogged up with a collection of waste and corruption.

This is one particular angle of the problem of nutrition which is generally overlooked. I refer to the elimination from the system of waste matter from the colon.

It is impossible, when we eat two, three or more meals a day, not to have residue accumulating in the colon in the form of undigested food particles as well as the end product from food which has undergone digestion.

Furthermore, not only does food-waste accumulate in the colon, but so do also the millions of cells and tissues which have served their purpose and have been replaced in the process of replenishment. These cells and tissues are dead proteins of a highly toxic nature if allowed to ferment and putrefy. You no doubt have experienced the offensive aroma emanating from the body of an animal which has died and whose carcass has begun to decompose. The cells and tissues in the anatomy undergo the same decomposition under favorable conditions, and the conditions are favorable when they are allowed to remain in the colon longer than necessary.

The very purpose of the colon as an organ of ELIMINATION is to collect all fermentative and putrefactive toxic waste from every part of the anatomy, and by the peristaltic waves of the muscles of the colon to remove all solid and semi-solid waste from the body.

In simple words, the colon is the sewage system of the anatomy. Nature's laws of preservation and hygiene require and insist that this sewage system be cleansed regularly, under penalty of the innumerable ailments, sickness and diseases that follow, as the night the day, if waste is allowed to accumulate.

Have you seen and studied the Chart that I made, entitled: COLON THERAPY CHART? It is a Chart measuring about 17 by 22 inches which can be framed and hung on the wall of your home or office, so your family, friends and clients can start thinking about their anatomy. Part of this Chart is reproduced herewith. It displays the shape of what the natural colon should look like. This is only one half of the Chart. On the other half, next to the "perfect" colon, I show six vignettes taken from X-rays of the colons of six of my students. These are truly frightful to contemplate, but OH! they are so instructive and revealing! The first expression that comes from people who see and examine these vignettes is: "Oh my! could it be possible that MY colon looks like that?"

This cleansing is being effectively carried on in homes by means of a regular rubber enema bag and a 30 inch number 22 rectal or colon tube. Detailed outlines of this procedure are given in my books *BECOME YOUNGER* and in the 1970 Edition of *FRESH VEGE-TABLE AND FRUIT JUICES, What's Missing in Your Body?* In these books you will also learn about the use and value of colon irrigations.

Not to cleanse the colon is like having the entire garbage collecting staff in your city go on strike for days on end! The accumulation of garbage in the streets creates putrid odoriferous unhealthy gases dispersed into the atmosphere. The fermentation and putrefaction of accumulated waste and corruption in the colon creates equally noxious gases which are not always expelled as they should be.

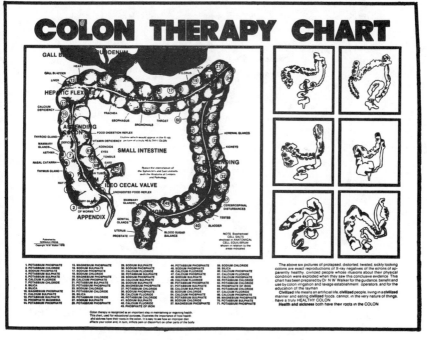

HOW NERVES OF THE COLON
AFFECT EVERY PART OF THE ANATOMY

When you realize that every pouch or sacculation of the colon is equipped with nerve terminals originating in every part of the anatomy, with definite and specific relation to the nerves of every unit of the glandular system, you will find it very revealing to study the accompanying sketches and to consider seriously the following paragraphs.

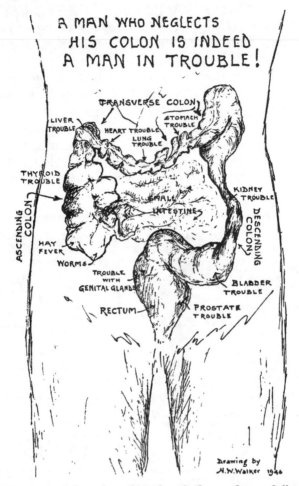

A MAN WHO NEGLECTS HIS COLON IS INDEED A MAN IN TROUBLE!

Drawing by N.W.Walker 1946

For example, the sketch of the colon of "A Man In Trouble" is the copy of an X-ray of an intelligent and educated chemist with whom I was very well acquainted, but who ridiculed every suggestion I made advising him to clean out his system and change his diet to the "Walker Program". "No, he would say, God made all foods for man to eat and I will go on eating all foods that appeal to me as long as I live". Well,—you guessed it. He died at the age of 45. You will enjoy reading the two pages **40 and 41** in my book BECOME YOUNGER. It details graphically just what happened to him, and why.

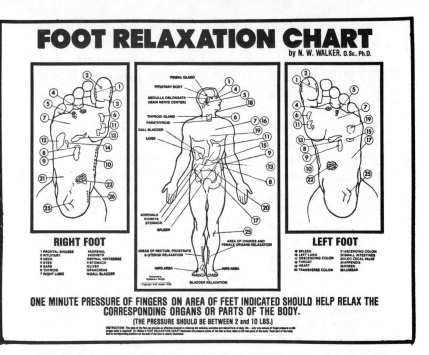

To the uninformed it sounds ridiculous to claim that there is a relation and co-relation between nerves in one part of the body and another remote part of the anatomy. Nevertheless this happens to be the case. The FOOT RELAXATION CHART (which also measures about 17 by 22 inches) which I have made, clearly shows the lines of the relative communication between the foot, particularly the soles of the feet, with other parts of the anatomy from head to foot, through the nerve system.

The treatment to help relieve many bodily disturbances by exerting finger-pressure on the sole of the feet has now become an accepted therapy. It is known as ZONE THERAPY.

WHAT CONSTITUTES NUTRITION?

The world's most serious problem is undoubtedly malnutrition. Civilized Nations are definitely as much afflicted with malnutrition as the most abject Nations living under starvation or near-starvation conditions, and this civilized phenomenon exists in spite of the fact that in civilization there is a superabundance of food.

The trouble stems from the fact that civilization feeds itself on the principle of palatability and under the cloud and snare of advertising indoctrination. Too much of

13

the food consumed in this day and generation is deficient in some of the most vital and essential elements.

The most vital nutritional element, of course, is the ENZYMES which constitute the life principle in every atom and molecule composing every LIVE organism. Besides being present and active in raw vegetation, Enzymes are present and involved in the human anatomy and in all its activities and functions.

Enzymes are sensitive to high temperatures. Up to about 125°F they are at the peak of their efficiency and are no less alive at temperatures of 50 and 60 degrees below zero. When they are subject to a temperature of 130°F they are destroyed. They are DEAD.

Obviously when food is cooked, or at any rate when it is heated at temperatures above 130°F, no live Enzymes are left in it. It has become dead food.

Naturally dead matter cannot do the work of live organisms, consequently food which has been subjected to temperatures above 130°F has lost its live nutritional value. While such food can, and does, sustain life in the human system it does so at the expense of progressively degenerating health, energy and vitality.

This state of affairs is graphically observed when a farmer tries to feed pasteurized milk to a calf. Pasteurized milk is heated at a temperature high enough supposedly to destroy pathogenic bacteria. While doing so it also kills all Enzymes in the milk. Calves fed on pasteurized milk have died within six months!

Every plant, vegetable, fruit, nut and seed in its raw natural state is composed of atoms and molecules, every single one of these being replete with Enzymes. Atoms and molecules composing the human anatomy correspond to, and are in sympathetic relationship with those in the food we eat. The object and purpose of NUTRITION is to replenish and regenerate the atoms and molecules composing the cells and tissues in the body.

In the course of the voluntary and involuntary activities of the body we expend considerable unconscious energy. This energy is furnished by the Enzymes in the atoms in the cells and tissues. When, in this process, the Enzymes have carried out their function, the atoms involved are discarded, they are automatically passed into the blood and lymph streams and are transferred into the colon for expulsion as waste.

14

As soon as such atoms are expended they are replaced by corresponding atoms obtained from the food eaten, constantly carrying on the cycle of replenishment and regeneration. It is on the quality of this replacement that we build up health, energy and vitality — or the reverse.

It is obvious, on this fact, on this premise and on this basis that sickness, disease and premature old age cannot be other than the result of our failure to nourish our body with the food and nourishment which will regenerate, revitalize and reanimate the cells and tissues of our anatomy, of our glands in particular and of our bloodstream, nerve and muscle systems in general.

The mysterious operation of our digestive system takes place by virtue of the Enzymes which are present in every live atom and molecule composing the cells and tissues of the body and consequently in all the performances and functions of the human system.

In the constitution of the human anatomy there are strange and intricate laboratories in which ultramicroscopic vital substances are generated. These laboratories form the ENDOCRINE GLAND system. These vital substances are known as hormones which trickle directly into the bloodstream by the process of osmosis as there is no duct or outlet for them otherwise to be collected by the blood. It is the presence of Enzymes throughout each gland that makes this transfer possible.

The most important component of these hormones, besides their Enzymes, is the number of rare infinitesimal microscopic TRACE ELEMENTS indiscernible, imperceptible and invisible except by means of extremely powerful microscopes or other highly scientific instruments.

Until comparatively recently these trace elements were not even recognized. Today we know that there are at least 43 of these trace elements in addition to the 16 elements which compose the main structure of matter.

We therefore know today that there are at least 59 elements in the constitution of the human anatomy and its functions and activities, and we also know that any lack or unbalance of any one or more of them has a direct bearing on the health and sickness that assails humanity.

A list of these trace elements is given in my book *FRESH VEGETABLE AND FRUIT JUICES, What's*

Missing in Your Body? in the 1970 Edition, and I need not repeat it here. It is of vital importance, however, that these be kept replenished and in balance in the system, constantly. Consequently, we should eat a sufficient variety of the foods that contain most of these, raw and fresh, every day, if we expect to maintain a fairly evenly balanced and healthy body.

In my family (of two) we try to eat daily two or three of the following foods which contain more or less virtually all the 59 elements, namely:

Alfalfa, Beets, Cabbage, Capsicum, Carrots, Corn, Cucumbers, Leaf Dulse, Filberts (Hazel Nuts), Jerusalem Artichokes, Kelp, Mung Beans, Olives, (dried), Papayas, Pignolias (Pine Nuts), Pumpkin Seeds and Watercress.

I must point out, however, that hybrid plants are quite deficient in trace elements, particularly corn, and we avoid eating hybrid foods, whenever possible.

Of course all other foods not listed here do contain trace elements, but usually in lesser quantities so that by eating plenty of all available fresh raw vegetables and fruits, and particularly drinking their juices, we can be fairly certain that we are getting our complement of the trace and other elements which the system requires.

One item which we consider invaluable and indispensable is SEA or OCEAN WATER. We use the CATALINA SEA WATER which we can obtain from the Health Food Stores. This is taken from the Pacific Ocean many miles west of the California Coast beyond Catalina Island. We have found it to be live, organic water containing all of the 59 elements. We use just about a quarter of a teaspoon of this to a full glass of whatever we are drinking, and we add this also to our salads.

One word of warning — however — DO NOT USE the water which comes from any inland salt water sea or lake. We have found that such water is not beneficial. On the contrary, it may cause disturbances in the system.

SEEDS

Seeds are a primary food. If it were possible to visualize the materialization of a Cosmic Concept, we would have the composite picture of a seed. The seed contains in its embryonic condition the entire pattern of the atoms, molecules, cells and tissues that will appear as its plant when fully grown.

In its natural, untreated, unprocessed form a seed is replete with enzymes. It is composed of proteins, carbohydrates and fats which can very easily be digested when properly prepared, either by sprouting or by grinding them very finely.

If a seed will sprout it proves that it is filled with the essence of Cosmic Life, alive with the very Breath of the Creator, God Almighty.

All the life giving elements necessary for the proper maintenance and propagation of life are sealed in the tiny seeds and they are created for the good and benefit of humanity.

Every chemical and mineral element which the vegetable, the plant and the tree contains was present in its full capacity in the fertile seed. So vitally important are seeds in the completeness of nutrition that we should try to have some every day in some form or another. However, seeds are a concentrated food and should be eaten in small amounts at a time. Seeds furnish more actual constructive nourishment than meat, and they are compatible with all foods, particularly when sprouted. All seeds and their sprouts are among the richest sources of protein, and also are rich in calcium and magnesium.

Hybrid seeds should be avoided as their constitutional balance has been interfered with detrimentally and their nutritional value has consequently been impaired. It is better to purchase seeds from a Health Food Store, or from some reputable person who grows them organically.

SPROUTING SEEDS

We try to serve fresh sprouted seeds at one or more meals every day. Our standby sprouts are Alfalfa, Mung Beans and sometimes Lentils. However, you can experiment on your own and find out what you like best, and thereby supplement your diet with much variety and added nutrition.

There are many gadgets sold for sprouting seeds, but we still like a wide mouth glass Mason Fruit Jar best of all. If you want to sprout a small amount of seeds you can use the one quart size, but the 2-quart size is more practical. Some of the Health Food Stores are now selling a 2-quart wide mouth Kerr Mason glass fruit jar with a special lid, the center of which is a plastic screen fastened tightly to the rim which screws on the top of the jar to replace the regular lid — it is called "SPROUT-EASY". The instructions for using it are fastened to one side of the jar. If you cannot find these jars, you can use the regular wide mouth Kerr Mason fruit jars — which you should be able to buy at any Supermarket — using a piece of either fine or coarse Nylon net over the top of the jar fastening it on tightly with the outer rim. Then when the sprouts are ready to eat you can replace this with the regular inside removable metal rim and store them in the refrigerator until they have all been used up. This white Nylon net can be purchased in the yardage section of almost any Department Store and the price is very reasonable. It is easy to wash and keep clean and it can be used over and over again.

For either Alfalfa or Mung Bean sprouts we use 2-tblsp of seeds which we have purchased at the Health Food Store and which are guaranteed to sprout. Prepare the seeds by measuring them out on a large plate and remove all broken seeds, as these will not sprout, and any bits of gravel which you may find in them. Then pour the seeds into a fine mesh tea strainer and wash them thoroughly by running cold water through them from the tap. Pour the 2-tblsp of Mung Beans into one quart jar and the 2-tblsp of Alfalfa seeds into a 2-quart jar, add one pint of tepid water to each, cover and let set overnight to soak.

Next morning put on the lid with the screen, or fasten a piece of Nylon net over the top of each jar and drain off the water, rinse once in cool water, drain off ALL the water and put the jar on its side either on a plate or tray, shaking the seeds around to distribute them as evenly as possible on the lower side of the jar.

Each day keep a close watch on them to be sure that they do not dry out — they must be kept moist in order for them to sprout. Usually rinsing twice daily is sufficient, but four or five times may be necessary during the hot weather in hot climates. Where there is a lot of humidity in the atmosphere they may have a tendency to mold, but after you have experimented a while you will find out what method is best for your climate and circumstances.

Small seeds take longer to sprout, therefore it may take 4 or 5 days for Alfalfa sprouts to be ready to use, while in two or three days Mung Bean sprouts are ready. When they have reached the size you like best, lay the jars in full sunlight in front of a window if possible and keep turning them at intervals until each side shows little green leaves on the sprouts. Then they can be rinsed two or three times in cold water, thoroughly drained, tightly covered and stored in the refrigerator until crisp —and they are delicious. We believe some fresh air needs to get into the seeds as they are sprouting, so we do not put them away in a dark closet or cupboard but leave them setting out in the open in the kitchen, merely covering the glass part of the jar with paper towels or a clean tea towel to keep out excessive light. This speeds up the growth of the sprouts.

As soon as one batch of sprouts is stored in the refrigerator you can start another, and in this way keep a constant supply of fresh green ones coming up. They should be used as soon as possible, for if left too long in the refrigerator they lose their flavor. We try to use them up within 4 or 5 days. Experience will guide you in the quantity your family will consume and how often you need to sprout more seeds.

These are delicious mixed in any salad, eaten just as they are or finely chopped up in a salad. They also serve as a nice garnish for the top of a salad. These sprouts give much substance and added nourishment to an all-raw food meal, and are particularly good for a growing family.

SEED AND NUT MILKS
We use Seed and Nut Milks instead of cream or milk. The following is our favorite recipe:

Put the following into the bowl of one of the little electric nut and seed grinders which can be obtained from your Health Food Store — (Moulinex or any other make).

    2 — tbsp Raw shelled Sunflower seeds

   12 — Whole raw Almonds with skin on,

    1 — tbsp Whole Sesame seeds.

Grind to a very fine powder then put it in your Blender

with 1-pint of warm water and 1-tbsp of mild honey and thoroughly blend at high speed for 2 or 3 minutes. This is then ready to serve over your breakfast.

This is the basic recipe and it can be varied according to your taste. If you want it richer and more like thick cream, use less water, and you can use more or less honey according to the way you like it best. If you want it thinner and less rich, add more water.

This is delicious over a breakfast of sliced bananas, soaked black Mission figs and soaked Thompson seedless raisins, triturated fresh carrot pulp and Mung Bean sprouts. Over this can be sprinkled a combination of Sunflower and Pumpkin seeds with raw Almonds ground together to a meal in the little electric nut and seed grinder. A large glass of carrot juice with this gives a nourishing breakfast to satisfy even a hard working man.

HOW AND WHY
TO EAT CORRECTLY

To the uninformed, it may appear that too much stress is placed on the loss of the nourishing value of the vegetables and fruits when they are cooked.

The purpose of the suggestions contained herein is not to advocate eating only raw foods, nor necessarily to give up the food we like most, but rather to enable everyone desirous of doing so, to give a fair prolonged trial to the regime of diet that has reduced fatigue and restored energy, vigor and vitality to a great many people.

These suggestions are published at the repeated request of many of the thousands of people who have attended my lectures on the subject. They have urged me to publish an outline of the diet and menus which I have followed rigidly for years, and to which I attribute the indefatigable energy which I have enjoyed by adhering strictly to this method of eating.

I do not advocate, nor as a general rule do I recommend, changing from the customary eating habits completely and suddenly. The reaction from doing so, while generally constructive and cleansing to the body, may cause more discomfort temporarily than is desired or anticipated.

If will power and fortitude are strong enough attributes, coupled with the individual's determination to give Nature every ounce possible of cooperation, surprisingly satisfactory results will follow.

Unfortunately we have become a race seeking pain-killing remedies for instant relief, disregarding consequences, rather than choosing ways to eradicate the cause of our bodily discomforts by means of the slower and more tedious, but decidedly more certain and permanent methods of aiding Nature to cleanse, rebuild and regenerate the body in order that our life may be longer, more vital and consequently more useful.

Insomnia for example is one of the afflictions daily becoming more pernicious among Americans with the result that sedatives and sleeping pills of all kinds, invariably containing drugs, are finding a daily increasing demand. Any drug that induces sleep cannot be anything but habit-forming, advertisements to the contrary notwithstanding, because if the habit is not physical then it becomes mental. Inability to sleep is due to malnutrition and toxic conditions in the body reacting on the nerve system so that the individual loses the power to induce sleep while that condition exists.

Many sleeping-pill drug addicts have found that a large tumbler full of fresh grapefruit juice before going to bed at night, and a high enema to clean out the lower intestines, have helped them to the point where they were able to sleep without the use of pills or powders, with a little change in their diet. Others have found that a glassful of straight celery juice or lettuce juice worked as efficiently when these juices were properly extracted and taken fresh and raw. A change in the diet is usually more beneficial when concentrated sugars and starches are eliminated.

I am firmly convinced that there is an ever-increasing demand for this knowledge. It is so extremely simple, and yet as old as the hills. More and more people are awakening to the fact that seeking the aid of Nature is more to be desired than blind guessing. After all, except in the case of accident, very little can happen to our body except as a result of what we put into it.

HOW TO COMBINE FOODS

With few exceptions I have found that raw fruits and vegetables are perfectly compatible when eaten together, either mixed in a salad or separately during the same meal.

Melons of all kinds should be eaten alone, the whole meal consisting of nothing but melon.

Fruits are the cleansers of the body. Their higher carbon content acts somewhat as an incinerator of debris in the system. Vegetables on the other hand are the builders of the body, containing a somewhat higher relative proportion of protein and a somewhat smaller proportion of carbon, or carbohydrates.

Fruits should only be eaten when they are ripe, because until they are ripe the sugars have not formed completely and therefore will have an acid reaction in the system. Ripe fruit, although apparently acid to the taste, has an alkaline reaction in the body.

It is extremely important to bear in mind that if refined sugar of any kind whatsoever, or any flour product in any form or manner, is eaten during the same meal with fruits (except bananas, dates, figs or raisins) either together or within an hour or two, the sugars and starches will have a tendency to ferment in the digestive tract and sooner or later a chemical reaction, frequently called acidosis, or an acidulated condition of the stomach, is likely to result.

A study of the Food Chart will assist in choosing foods so that they may be combined in a compatible manner.

HOW TO KNOW WHAT TO EAT AND HOW TO LIVE

The fundamental purpose of eating is to replenish the chemical elements composing the cells and tissues in our body. Replenishment is one of the basic laws of Nature in regard to organic chemistry, and our physical body is a laboratory functioning under organic chemistry principles.

The food that we eat should nourish these cells and tissues. Unfortunately, because Nature gave to man a body so elastic, so far as taking punishment is concerned, that it can survive for years on food which is destructive to the body, but appealing to his appetite and palate, man has indulged these appetites until the race is perceptibly degenerating mentally, as well as physically.

The body is the vehicle of the mind, and the mind is the vehicle of the intellect. The intellect is that part of the mind that we use in observing and reasoning.

If the body is permitted to degenerate, then the intellect cannot be expected to function or develop constructively, as the spiritual and mental faculties in man grow and expand in direct relation to the improvement, regeneration and purity of the physical body.

We look on sickness and disease as something mysterious and dreadful and we blame germs and bacteria.

As a matter of fact germs and bacteria are the scavengers of Nature and are everywhere. When we breathe, we inhale millions of these little natural scavengers and it is their function to keep the debris in our body neutralized and to stir it up so that it can be eliminated from the body. It is *our* job, however, to keep our body in such condition that this elimination can be completed to perfection.

Due to the excessive quantity of inorganic food that we eat, food in which the life principle has been destroyed by cooking, canning, and other processes, this debris, or end-product of the digestion of this food, in the body, accumulates faster than we and these natural scavengers can remove it. The result is that germs and bacteria find a feeding ground within us in which to propagate. In this process of their propagation the sewage of their colonies is added to the debris and the result is what we call sickness or disease.

Whenever germs and bacteria enter a body which is thoroughly clean and healthy, within and without, they find no feeding ground of waste or morbid matter therein on which to colonize and therefore pass out of the system in the natural course of events.

Likewise, when all debris and accumulated morbid matter is removed from a sick or diseased body, then only is established the first step toward a recovery to a normal chemical balance.

How does this debris and morbid matter get into the body? In two distinct ways.

First, through the food, etc., which is eaten to excess in inorganic form cooked, etc., which can neither be assimilated by the body for constructive purposes, nor be properly eliminated; and also by such unnatural elements as serums, vaccines, injections, etc. These cause deposits which the body is unable to throw off in the course of its normal functions, if the eliminative channels are in any way impaired.

Second, through the cells and tissues of the body which in the course of our activities are constantly used up and remain there as dead matter after furnishing physical and mental energy. These used-up cells should leave the body as soon as possible after they have served their function, but they remain in the system for unnecessarily long periods of time due to faulty elimination.

We can give here only briefly a few of the interesting reasons why nourishing the body properly is of such vital importance. A brief outline of the process that causes the greatest accumulation of debris in the body is necessary so that we may be guided intelligently in the selection and combination of our foods.

Let us take, for example, an individual, 40 years of age. Undoubtedly like the majority of his fellow men he has formed the habit of eating at least three meals a day. This will average more than 1,000 meals a year, or in excess of 40,000 meals during his lifetime of 40 years. It is very important that we bear this in mind.

We will also assume that, like most people, nearly all the food he has eaten has been cooked, canned or otherwise processed, and rarely, if ever, does he eat either a sufficient quantity of raw food, or a complete meal of nothing but raw vegetables and fruits. The result therefore is that more than 40,000 meals, composed mostly of dead food (or inorganic chemical elements) have passed through his system during that time.

It is impossible to regenerate organic cells in a human body with inorganic (or dead) matter. We find that while the 40,000 meals did serve the purpose of *sustaining* life, hardly any nourishment in organic form was eaten to regenerate the cells and tissues of his body or supply the chemical elements composing these.

As a matter of fact it is appalling to realize that the limit of tolerance of such a condition is usually reached by the time we are 40 or 50 years of age, an age at which mature judgment and experience have been gained, a period in life when we should know what life has in store for us, the very prime of life, but the age at which most men and women find themselves with a neglected body which is degenerating rapidly and is no longer an efficient vehicle in which to put that knowledge and experience into practical use, speedily heading for premature senility and the discard.

We know that the body requires bulk. The error in judgment is in the interpretation of what function the bulk is intended to perform. To be of any value whatever, the bulk in our food must be composed of the raw cellulose, or fiber, of raw vegetables and fruits eaten as nearly as possible in their natural ripe state.

When so eaten, after proper mastication, the digestive processes extract as many as possible of the chemical elements contained in the fibers. The remaining bulk goes through the intestines becoming, figuratively speaking, highly magnetized by means of the muscular kneading of their peristaltic action. Thus they draw into the intestines from every part of the body the used-up cells and tissues, eliminating these, as well as the debris resulting from normal digestion and the end-products thereof, through the colon, thereby acting both as an intestinal broom and as a vacuum cleaner.

When food has been cooked or processed in any manner or form, however, the fiber or cellulose is converted into an inorganic substance in which every vestige of life has been destroyed. The fiber being lifeless therefore can no longer work as a broom or as a vacuum cleaner, but operates instead like a mop (usually a slimy one) pushing matter along without any cleansing effect. Due to lack of magnetic attraction, which cannot be generated in dead fiber, it has no ability whatsoever to draw into the intestines used up cells and tissues from other parts of the body, nor any other toxic matter which may have accumulated therein.

Consider these two pictures. On the one hand an abundance of raw fibers passing through the digestive and eliminative tracts, acting as a cleansing broom and as a vacuum cleaner after every meal, three times a day, leaving not only a clean intestinal tract each time but also removing from the system other accumulated waste matter. On the other hand visualize the bulk, or fiber of cooked, devitalized food (nearly always in excessive quantities) passing through the intestines and eliminative organs three times a day—40,000 times or more in 40 years—every time leaving a coating of slime. 40,000 coatings of slime, be they ever so thin, are bound to leave their mark.

Man is the only member of the animal kingdom who, notwithstanding his supposedly higher intelligence, indulges his appetites at the expense of his body, and pampers these deliberately, without using common sense or good judgment, listening to the silky voice of deception telling him that food has nothing to do with the condition of his body.

With such a microscopic use of our intelligence it is not surprising that just when we have reached the age when our knowledge and experience are of value to us, for us to use to advantage, and we are really anxious to begin to LIVE, we find ourselves handicapped with a physical body which is ready for the discard, if not for the grave.

The problem therefore is to know how to change our eating habits to regenerate our body, without too much discomfort, and reactions too strong for the comfort of the mind or the vicissitudes of our daily life, and what will enable us to achieve eventually a healthy body free from fatigue, sickness and disease.

It is interesting to note that the public and its educators are just now beginning to realize the value of, and talking a great deal about "preventive medicine," a subject which I have proved and preached from practical experience for more than a quarter of a century.

The first step is internal cleanliness. A thorough, and, to begin with, a continual daily cleansing of the lower intestines is imperative. The high enema has proved invaluable in this respect. A very good description of this is given in the detoxication chapter of the book *FRESH VEGETABLE AND FRUIT JUICES* by N. W. Walker, D.Sc., and *BECOME YOUNGER* by N. W. Walker, D.Sc.

For quicker results, a better and more thorough internal cleansing is obtained by means of colonic irrigations properly used and administered. I have found the most satisfactory results were obtained when four or five irrigations were taken on consecutive days, one each day. These were followed by one, two or three weekly thereafter.

If properly administered with the right kind of equipment I have found these extremely beneficial with no discomfort whatever.

Those who have never taken them are not qualified to, nor capable of, giving an opinion that is of any value whatsoever. Advice against colonic irrigations with the proper kind of equipment intelligently administered, cannot come from anyone unless he is utterly ignorant of the first and fundamental principles of body cleanliness.

The reason or excuse given that they are weakening and therefore harmful, is absolute nonsense. The ulterior motive for such reasoning is purely and simply lack of knowledge and experience. This subject is covered in detail in the book *BECOME YOUNGER* by N. W. Walker, D.Sc.

As a matter of fact, the colon is the cesspool of the body. How can the body recover strength and its proper chemical balance, if this is not cleaned out first of all?

ATOMS COMPOSING THE VITAL CHEMICALS IN THE BODY

Our next consideration is to enable the law of replenishment to work in our body. The human body is not just like one of our business chemical laboratories, but a **vital chemical laboratory,** and is composed of practically all the atomic elements of the mineral kingdom, but in organic, vital, life-containing form. The most important of these atoms are given in the following list in approximately the proportions indicated.

THE ADULT HUMAN BODY
is composed on an average of the following atomic elements

Element	Approximate		Combines principally with	In the formation mainly of
	Per cent.	Quantity		
Oxygen	65	98 lbs.	Calcium Iron Sulphur Phosphorus	Bones, Teeth, Skin, Red Blood corpuscles, Circulation, Optimism.
Carbon	18	27 lbs.	Silicon Oxygen	Teeth, Connective Tissue Skin, Hair, Nails.
Hydrogen	10	15 lbs.	Oxygen Sodium Chlorine	Blood, and all the Cells in the body.
Nitrogen	3	4 lbs. 8 oz.	Potassium Chlorine	Muscles, Cartilage, Tissues, Ligaments, Tendons, lean flesh.

(continued on next page)

Calcium	2	3 lbs.	Carbon Oxygen	Bones and Teeth.
Phosphorus	1	1 lb. 8 oz.	Sodium Carbon Oxygen	Blood and Brains.
Potassium	0.4	9.6 oz.	Calcium Phosphorus Oxygen	Blood, Bones and all cells.
Sulphur	0.25	6 oz.	Potassium Carbon Oxygen	Blood.
Sodium	0.25	6 oz.	Calcium Sulphur Oxygen	Skin, Nerves, Mucous Membrane.
Chlorine	0.25	6 oz.	Nitrogen Sulphur Oxygen	Epithelium, Nerves, etc.
Fluorine	0.2	4.8 oz.	Potassium Sulphur Oxygen	Nails, Hair, Blood, Skin.
Magnesium	0.05	1.2 oz.	Potassium Hydrogen Phosphorus Oxygen	Blood, Nerves, Muscles.
Iron	0.008	0.2 oz.	Sodium Hydrogen Phosphorus Oxygen	Blood, Bones, Brain, Muscles, etc.
Manganese	0.003	0.075 oz.	Iron Oxygen Hydrogen	Hemoglobin, Lymph, etc.
Silicon	0.0002	Trace	Iron Phosphorus Oxygen	Blood, Muscles, Nerves, Skin, Nails, Hair.
Iodine	0.00004	Trace	Iron Magnesium Phosphorus Oxygen	Thyroid, Blood, Spinal Nerves, Brain, Bone, Metabolism.

The following foods, etc., rich in the indicated atomic chemical elements, are listed in the order of their importance in relation thereto.

Oxygen   Breathe deeply to obtain free oxygen and drink as much fresh raw juices of fruits and vegetables as possible to obtain organic oxygen.

Carbon   Nuts, especially unsalted almonds, but not peanuts—(peanuts are exceedingly acid-forming). —Nut butters are very good if raw but not when heated in any manner whatever. Olives and avocados (alligator pears) are excellent sources of carbon. Butter (unsalted) and cream are also good sources when not pasteurized.

Hydrogen   Carrots, celery, spinach, cabbage, lettuce, tomatoes, grapes, huckleberries, red raspberries.

Nitrogen   Breathe deeply and rhythmically in open spaces. Alfalfa and other green leafy vegetables.

Calcium   Almonds (unsalted), carrots, dandelions, turnips, spinach, oranges, goat's milk (raw) for infants, okra, cauliflower, tomatoes, garlic, parsnips, all berries, all nuts (except peanuts), apples, potatoes (raw), apricots.

Phosphorus   Kale, radishes (large white), asparagus, sorrel, watercress, Brussels sprouts, garlic, Savoy cab-

28

	bage, carrots, cauliflower, squash, cucumbers, leeks, lettuce, turnips, Brazil nuts, walnuts, huckleberries, blackberries, cherries, black Mission figs, oranges, limes.
Potassium	Carrots, celery, parsley, spinach, beets, cauliflower, leeks, garlic, raw potatoes, sorrel, squash, tomatoes, turnips, oranges, lemons, apricots, bananas, cherries, dates, grapes, huckleberries, figs, pears, peaches, plums, raspberries, watermelon, pomegranate, olives.
Sulphur	Brussels sprouts, watercress, kale, horseradish, cauliflower, cabbage, chives, garlic, sorrel, cranberries, raspberries, pineapple, currants, apples, Brazil nuts, filberts.
Sodium	Celery, carrots, spinach, tomatoes, strawberries, radishes, squash, lettuce, dandelion, leeks, cucumbers, beets, turnips, apples, apricots, watermelon, huckleberries, pears, oranges, grapefruit, lemons, dates, cherries, grapes.
Chlorine	Beets, cabbage, celery, garlic, horseradish, parsnips, sweet potatoes, tomatoes, avocado, dates, pomegranate, cocoanut.
Fluorine	Almonds (unsalted), carrots, beet tops, turnip tops, dandelion, spinach, celery tops, goats milk (raw), Swiss cheese, egg yolks (beat up raw with honey in orange juice), cauliflower, cabbage, watercress, parsley, cucumber.
Magnesium	Carrots, celery, cucumbers, almonds (unsalted), dandelions, garlic, leeks, kale, lettuce, tomatoes, spinach, lemons, oranges, apples, blackberries, bananas, figs, pineapple, Brazil nuts, pecans, pinons, walnuts.
Iron	Lettuce, leeks, carrots, dandelions, radishes, asparagus, turnips, cucumbers, horseradish, tomatoes, almonds (unsalted), avocado, strawberries, raisins, figs, watermelon, apricots, cherries, huckleberries, walnuts, Brazil nuts, apples, grapes (Concord particularly), pineapple, oranges.
Manganese	Parsley, carrots, celery, beets, cucumbers, chives, watercress, almonds (unsalted), apples, apricots, walnuts.
Silicon	Cucumbers, lettuce, parsnips, asparagus tips (raw), beet tops, dandelion, horseradish, leeks, okra, parsley, green peppers, radishes, spinach, watercress, strawberries, cherries, apricots, apples, watermelon, figs.
Iodine	Kelp, sea lettuce, carrots, Irish moss, pineapple. (Note: Do not use medicated or liquid iodine as a food or drink.)

VITAMINS.   Much as the layman likes to play with mysterious subjects, Vitamin information in general is of little value to him unless he is familiar with the physiology of nutritional vitality and of his body. The inter-relation of the Vitamins with the proportions of the chemical elements in our foods forms a very complex subject which in most cases leaves the student in a web of confusion, unless he follows the study through, systematically.

Many foods contain all of the elements required by the body—such as oatmeal and other cereals, for example,—yet these are present in such proportions and combinations that in the process of human digestion their use actually has a disintegrating effect, in the long run, whereas such grains, fed to cattle, whose digestion is able completely to digest the concentrated starches and proteins, enables them to thrive on it.

For this reason I prefer to advise giving less concentrated thought to Vitamins and Vitamin problems and more attention to the increase of raw vegetables and fruits and their fresh raw juices, a least until time can be given to their systematic study in conjunction with the other nutritional details with which they are inextricably woven.

By drinking plenty of fresh, properly extracted, raw vegetable juices, in sufficient variety, there is no danger to fear Vitamin deficiency in my experience.

WATER

The processes of digestion are vital processes in which water, organic water, plays by far the most important part. The digestive juices themselves in the body are composed of more than 98% organic water. In their operation it is important that this organic water be constantly replenished.

The average human being evaporates about one gallon of water during 24 hours.

Water is composed of chemical elements and the only way in which it can become organic, or in other words be instilled with the life-principle, is through the vegetable kingdom.

The chemicals of the mineral kingdom are dead and inorganic, but when dissolved by Nature and absorbed in plant life, or vegetation, then they become organized with the life principle and so become organic.

The destruction of life in fruits and vegetables by means of fire, excessive heat or manufacturing processes, re-converts the organic chemicals back into their inorganic, lifeless state.

This applies equally to water. Whether it comes from the faucet, from the spring, from rain, or is distilled, water is inorganic; when fed to vegetation it is absorbed into the plant and becomes organic. The elements composing the original water are then separated and stored in the fibers of the plant. Therefore *the raw juice from all fruits and vegetables is the finest organic water obtainable.*

In the extraction of this water, as juice, we find also in it the other chemicals that were in the vegetable or fruit, and in this natural state these also are organic.

CARBOHYDRATES—PROTEINS

The human body is a *vital* organism and the digestion and assimilation of food takes place by means of *vital* **processes.** Destructive fermentation and putrefaction in the body result from eating at the same time combinations of foods containing concentrated sugar and starch carbohydrates with those containing concentrated proteins, or with acid fruits.

All vegetables and fruits, when raw, contain all of the carbohydrate sugars and the proteins required by the body. These are present in very minute but ample quantities, while water is present in a relatively abundant volume.

Nearly all vegetables and fruits contain, when fresh and raw, from 50% to as high as 95% or more water. The carbohydrate and protein content ranges from a fraction of 1% to, in a few cases, as high as 10%.

When fed in proper combinations the body can be and is perfectly nourished by means of a diet consisting solely of raw vegetables and fruits, and nuts, supplemented by a sufficient quantity of freshly and properly made raw vegetable and fruit juices.

Due to the presence of a correspondingly large quantity of water in raw vegetables and fruits, these may be eaten together, when desired, in any combination, provided no sugar is used. Honey however is a natural carbohydrate and can be used with all or any food.

It has been my experience that once the body has been thoroughly cleansed and has become accustomed to such a regime for several months or years, the individual becomes indefatigable with an almost inexhaustible supply of energy, vigor and vitality, as well as an astonishing amount of strength and endurance. I am speaking here from personal experience, because I have repeatedly found that under such a regime the cells and tissues of the body are instantly replenished and regenerated whenever they are called upon to furnish energy, so that eventually fatigue is practically impossible.

In the final analysis fatigue is the inability of the cells of the body to replenish and regenerate fast enough to furnish continuously the energy they are called upon to give forth. Consequently fatigue is the first manifestation that the cells in the body are starved and are not regenerating quickly enough, even though an abundant volume of cooked food may have been ingested daily. It is the first indication that the body is heading for disease and sickness and eventual disintegration.

When food is cooked, canned or otherwise processed, then the sugars are converted into starches. The body actually has no means of using starches as such but must convert them into certain types of sugars to be able to use them. This adds to the work of the digestive organs. The claim that the body needs concentrated starches as a steady diet is utterly false.

Starch and sugar carbohydrates require an alkaline digestion. When used in concentrated form (such as in flour products of any kind, breads, cereals, sugars, candy, etc.), they should never be eaten during the same meal in which concentrated proteins (such as meats, eggs, milk, etc.), are included. These would result in incompatible chemical combinations, which would involve the destructive fermentation of the carbohydrates and the putrefaction of the proteins, creating an excessively acid condition.

Nor should concentrated carbohydrates ever be used with fruits of the acid or semi-acid kind, because the fruits would cause fermentation of the carbohydrates and, besides, they would then no longer have an alkaline reaction in the body, but on the contrary, would increase its acidity.

A study of the Food Chart on page 120 will show how, with a little practice, foods can easily be segregated, and by combining all foods consistently in the manner indicated a long step in the right direction will have been taken.

As a general rule I do not consider it advisable for most people to change their eating habits suddenly to a regime of only raw foods. It seems to me that it is sometimes better to make the change gradually, yet as quickly as possible, consistent with the conditions of the individual.

By eating raw foods only, excluding all cooked and processed foods, for one, two or three days a week, and, during the other days of the week carefully planning the meals so that every combination is absolutely compatible (in accordance with the Food Chart suggestions), drinking also one or two glasses of fresh raw vegetable juices at the beginning of every meal, whenever possible, it should take but a short while to adapt oneself to the change.

VEGETABLE AND FRUIT JUICES

The juices must be raw, freshly made, preferably by means of a triturating machine and hydraulic press. Long and costly experience have convinced me that this is the most satisfactory and practically the only way to extract *all* of the vitamins, enzymes and minerals from the vegetables.

I have found that one can drink, with much benefit, several pints of fresh raw vegetable juices daily when these are properly made. One pint a day seems to be the least that will show perceptible results. Any discomfort from drinking them is usually due to the stirring up of conditions in the body which Nature is anxious to help to clear up, and as soon as eliminated, an increase in vigor and energy usually follow.

It is invariably the case, without exception, that anyone disapproving of, or objecting to fresh raw vegetable juices, when properly extracted, does not know, from personal experience, enough about them or of their physiological effect on the cells and tissues and digestive system of the body, to be competent to give an opinion.

I am interested in the advertisement which has just come to me in the mail, of a pill and capsule manufacturer. It is a circular intended solely "for the profession" in which figures are given, as an example, of one particular doctor whose income from the sale of these capsules alone, to his patients, netted him considerably more than $20,000 in 6 years!

There is no drug in the world which can supply the blood stream with the nourishment which will rebuild and regenerate the human body. At best, drugs and medicine are temporary crutches. Raw vegetable juices however are neither medicine nor drugs. If fresh and properly extracted they are the most vital rebuilding and regenerating food which the body can have for constructive purposes and the quickest means by which the body can be brought back to a normal condition of proper chemical balance.

It is always well to bear in mind what the ulterior motive of the critic may be when he ridicules or objects to raw vegetable juices and to other natural foods and natural ways as a means to re-establish the chemical balance of the body. The use of the raw juices of vegetables and fruits which Nature has so abundantly furnished for us, is the surest and safest way, as well as the quickest, to nourish the starved cells of the body.

It is imperative that such juices be *raw—freshly made* in a thoroughly sanitary manner, and *properly extracted.*

Pasteurized or sterilized juices are of no value whatsoever for this purpose.

BREADS, CEREALS, CAKES
and other Starches

We have maintained for many decades that concentrated starches are incompatible in the human digestive assimilative processes.

Emphasis should be made that this fact applies to starch foods and products which have been subjected to heat in excess of 125°F. Excessive heat destroys the enzymes without which the cells and tissues of the body cannot be nourished and regenerated.

This applies to all foods and more particularly to starchy foods because in this day and generation starch has become the preeminent item in the food of the majority of civilized people.

Any contradictory claims to the contrary notwithstanding, the conclusive proof has been the improvement in the health of thousands of people whose diet was changed to drastically reduce, and preferably completely to eliminate all cooked starch foods and products.

The process which starts the breaking down of the starch molecules begins with the saliva in the mouth. The chemical process continues through the liver and the pancreas. It is when the final breakdown of the starch molecules reaches the tiny blood capillaries to transfer the end product of the broken-down starch molecule to the cells, that the real trouble begins.

The cooked product is lifeless. It has the tendency to clog up the microscopic capillaries leaving the expectant live cells and tissues to starve at the outlet of the capillaries.

There are many miraculous processes taking place constantly and continuously throughout the entire anatomy and all, without exception, are governed by inflexible Natural Laws.

You cannot have life and death at one and the same time. Consequently you cannot have a dead body, whether it be a dead molecule or a dead human being, carry on the activity requiring the life principle for its performance.

Under these circumstances it can be granted that cooked starches are digestible, as starch food advocates proclaim. But such is only a theoretical half-truth. Food merely digested has not yet served its purpose. It must go further. It must be capable of assimilation by the live active cells of the body. Only live foods, foods replete with enzymes from beginning to end, are capable of being assimilated at the final end of the digestive process.

It is only because Nature has instilled into the human system a colossal amount of tolerance for food which fails to nourish the vital cells, and also because there are such an astronomical number of cells, atoms and molecules in the system, to say nothing of the myriad of miles of tiny blood capillaries, that the human body is able to live as long as it does — or I should say is able to exist as long as it does, — in spite of the grievous, deplorable, onerous eating habits of most people.

The blood is the means by which nourishment reaches the cells and tissues of the body. The blood, however, is more than the mere transportation agent for food for the anatomy. Bear in mind that every drop of blood in the system makes from 3,000 to 5,000 round trips through the entire body every 24 hours. As the entire supply of blood in the human system amounts to about 5 quarts, and only 80% of this, or 4 quarts of blood, is in constant circulation, you must appreciate the need to watch meticulously what kind of molecules you allow to enter into it.

Once the food has been processed through the stomach and duodenum, the primary steps only have been achieved. From the duodenum onward, the blood is the main factor for the collection of the processed molecules. The blood cells, of which there are some 25,000,000,000 (twenty-five billion) in your body, do not have any selective ability. They are far too busy to waste time to choose any particular type or kind of molecule which you have put in your mouth, to do anything specific about it.

The blood cells just take what comes along, and the mysterious laws of magnetic attraction cause the molecules to be directed to their various processing stations along their way to their ultimate destination, which is the repair and regeneration of the cells and tissues of the anatomy.

This magnetic attraction is only available in live molecules for regenerative purposes. There are times and occasion when something goes amiss with a cell or a group of cells, when some element is needed to straighten things out. Such a condition is usually the precursor, the harbinger, the forerunner of an ailment or of sickness. Under such circumstances a catalyst is called for which need not necessarily be a "live" element, but it must be available in an infinitely microscopic molecular manner.

Grains can supply and make available such live elements when the grains are raw and have not been processed with poison sprays.

The molecules in cooked grains and their flours, as we have seen, are lifeless. The molecules of raw grains, including those of the shell and the germ and the entire grain, are replete with enzymes. The digestive processes, with their own enzymes, make the raw grain starch molecules available for cell regeneration, constructively, as well as becoming mere catalysts when called upon for such a purpose.

One can use raw grains beneficially. In their natural raw state grains are very hard, so just soak them in warm water (not over 125°F) in a large mouth Thermos bottle, overnight. By morning the hard shell is sufficiently softened to enable the grains to be easily ensalivated for processing further in the digestive system.

The grains we would recommend using are oats, rye and wheat, being careful to use only the organically grown unprocessed seeds, avoiding the commercial agricultural "treated" ones, such treatment being designed to prevent and destroy disease plant organisms.

Use just a small amount to begin with, say a scant teaspoonful. Remember that the first process of starch digestion begins in the mouth. Hold the grains in the mouth until they are thoroughly saturated with the saliva, then thoroughly chew them until liquefied before swallowing. Just take your time. If you have never tried this, I think it will be a revelation to you.

After becoming accustomed to this food for a few days, I expect you will be looking forward to this delicious item with which to start or to supplement your daily breakfast.

In my experience over many decades, as in the experience of a great many other investigators and people engaged in such research, breads, cakes, cereals and other cooked starchy foods can be blamed for a vast majority of the ailments that afflict today's civilization. I cannot emphasize too strongly that the best proof any one could want would be to try eliminating such foods for a few weeks, give the body a chance to rehabilitate itself and watch for unexpected if not unbelievable improvement.

MILK

It is generally assumed that cow's milk is one of our most perfect foods. A half truth is more misleading than a deliberate lie. Milk is the most mucus forming food in the human dietary, and from infancy to senility it is the most insidious cause of colds, flu, bronchial troubles, asthma, hay fever, pneumonia, tuberculosis and sinus trouble, according to our experience.

Milk is intended as food for the young, from birth until the skeletal bones and the rest of the anatomy is sufficiently developed for the assimilation of the natural foods required by the animal concerned. Thus cow's milk was never intended for a human infant. Nature meant it as nourishment for the calf.

A child's nutrition is natural when it is provided from its mother's milk. Such milk contains water, natural sugars, salts, amino acids, hormones, vitamins and the atoms of the elements necessary for the growth of the little body. One of the most important elements in milk is a substance called casein which furnishes a vast number of amino acids for the construction of the protein molecules building up the child's body. Casein is found only in milk and in eggs.

Cow's milk is vastly more coarse than mother's milk, and it contains 300% more casein than does mother's milk. Cow's milk is intended to double the weight of the calf in 6 to 8 weeks, whereas a child's body requires 6 to 7 months to double its weight. Cow's milk builds up the body structure of the calf to attain a weight of 1,000 to 2,000 lbs. at maturity. We have yet failed to find a man or woman whose ambition is the attainment of even 250 or 300 lbs. in weight!

Casein, by the way, is that material which is used to make the finest quality glue for woodwork. Cabinet makers use it extensively. Imagine what it does to the human system.

Another important consideration which is usually overlooked is the phosphorus content of milk. Phosphorus is one of the acid forming elements, and cow's milk contains almost 50% more phosphorus than is present in mother's milk. Furthermore the relation of the phosphorus to the sulphur content is disproportionate in these two kinds of milk, a most important consideration in regard to the mental and physical balance of the individual. The human body must exercise a vast amount of effort to metabolize cow's milk and the result of this effort, coupled with the inordinate amount of the casein content of the milk, is the cause of the mucous ailments which afflict humanity.

Raw cow's milk is bad enough—in view of the foregoing. However, to pasteurize milk and prescribe it for infants and invalids is, in my opinion and experience, incredible stupidity.

The pasteurization of milk originated when the

dairy industry degenerated into "big business." It is a practical impossibility to handle vast quantities of milk and milk products, transporting them long distances from place of origin to the large distributing centers, without considerable spoilage. Such spoilage, naturally, involves financial loss. The question of food value—live, organic atoms in the food—was subordinated to that of profits, and legislation was passed to protect such profits, without regard to the loss of the nourishment value of the food.

Unfortunately, the political machinery is still lubricated by mercenary instincts rather than by ethical integrity. If integrity were the rule, then the pasteurization of foods and the destruction of the life element or atoms in our food would receive closer attention and greater consideration. That, however, would involve such highly intelligent educational standards as would be beyond the comprehension of the politicians of today.

Suffice it to prove that the pasteurization of milk is no safeguard whatsoever for the health of the individual or of the community, and that it only prevents the milk from souring.

The claim that raw milk causes undulant fever and other diseases which would be prevented if it were pasteurized, is an utter and unmitigated falsehood. Pasteurization does *not* kill typhoid germs, nor bacilli coli, nor the germs of tuberculosis or of undulant fever.

In order to kill these pathogenic germs the milk would have to be heated to a temperature ranging all the way from 190° F. to 230° F. which would cause no cream to rise in the bottled milk—a great drawback from the merchandising viewpoint.

That pasteurized milk is unsafe and unfit for human consumption is proved by no less than 12 deaths in the city of San Francisco in 1928 attributed directly to pasteurized milk.

The year before, 1927, saw 5,002 cases of typhoid fever in the city of Montreal, Canada, with 533 deaths attributed directly to pasteurized milk.

Turning to our own records, we find that children of all ages, adolescents and adults invariably show incredible improvement when cow's milk has been omitted from the diet. Children who were perpetually afflicted with colds became healthier and stronger when fresh raw carrot and other juices were substituted for milk, and their colds disappeared.

Adults, afflicted with asthma, hay fever and other mucous conditions responded instantly to the elimination of milk from their diet, particularly when starches, also, were omitted.

The need for cow's milk as a necessary part of the human diet is purely and simply advertising propaganda with no foundation in fact. The recommendation of its use by any member of the healing profession is indicative of a lack of knowledge of the simple laws of the physiology of nutrition and lack of perception as to the fundamental cause of the presence of excessive mucus in the system.

There is not a member of the animal kingdom which uses milk as food after it has been weaned. It remains for man to develop such stupidity and to overlook the use of milk as the cause of so many of his ailments.

Nature placed the necessary ingredients in the milk of each type of animal, that were best suited for the growth of its young.

The fact that milk, used as a food after maturity, sustains life, is not disputed. Nor is the fact disputed that on rare occasions we find a goat nursing a calf, a bitch nursing kittens and a mare nursing pups. We even have records of a gorilla nursing a human child. These, however, are extreme natural emergencies and not habitual practices.

I have always maintained that education, from kindergarten through all the grades of school and college, should begin with and emphasize the study of the human anatomy and the physiology of nutrition. This means the science of life in our foods, the function of the living organism in vegetables and fruits in relation to the nourishment of the human body for the regeneration of its cells and tissues.

I also maintain that before a woman becomes pregnant, or immediately upon the realization that she is pregnant, she should study this subject to face intelligently the problems that lie ahead of her.

In the matter of her own nutrition, this now has a double function. Besides nourishing her own body so that her food can be more completely assimilated and her eliminative processes can function effectively, she also must furnish sufficient nourishment of the right kind for the efficient growth of the body of the child.

While it is true that milk contains a high percentage of calcium, an element essential in such a condition, nevertheless the other elements which constitute milk are so much out of balance in relation to the needs of the human body that they virtually destroy what benefits might otherwise accrue from the calcium. If the milk is pasteurized, that would be sufficient reason to avoid it altogether. Pasteurized milk used by mothers during pregnancy is probably the primary cause for the loss of their teeth, when little or no raw food and vegetable juices are used.

The calcium as well as all the other essential elements needed by the mother and the unborn child are found in raw vegetables and fruits, but to obtain them in sufficient quantity these must be supplemented by fresh raw vegetable juices. Carrot juice, for example, and carrot and spinach juice. (Study carefully the book *FRESH VEGETABLE AND FRUIT JUICES, What's Missing in Your Body?*)

The newborn child needs mother's milk. If this is not available, then the milk nearest to the chemical composition of mother's milk is goat's milk. This, however, should not be pasteurized, nor should it be heated to a greater temperature than 96° F., which is body temperature. After the first 3 or 4 weeks, carrot juice, freshly made, may be added to it with much benefit to the child. To begin with, one quarter carrot juice to three-quarters goat's milk, gradually increasing the quantity of carrot juice; this has proved very effective.

Soy and other legume milks have come into use of recent years. Because these are not animal products, the belief has grown that they are a good substitute for milk. The effect of soy bean products on the human digestion is definitely acid, notwithstanding the fact that in laboratory chemical tests an alkaline reaction may be obtained. As we are discussing these products in relation to milk, a brief comparison of soy milk with human and cow's milk may be quite enlightening.

Human milk is composed of about 87% organic water, cow's milk almost as much, while soy bean contains only little more than 10%. The addition of water in preparing soy flour into milk does not convert it into organic water. Human milk contains a little more than 1½% protein, cow's milk a little more than 3½% whereas soy bean milk is composed of more than 33% protein. Human milk contains a little more than 6% carbohydrates in the form of natural sugars, cow's milk nearly 5%, while soy milk is composed of more than 33% starchy carbohydrates. Human milk contains nearly 4% fat, cow's milk a little more than 3½%, while soy milk contains nearly 17% fat.

In relation to the chemical composition of human milk and soy milk, we find that the latter contains about 175% more phosphorus, about 400% more sulphur than does human milk, both these elements being acid forming. On the other hand, human milk contains about 3,500% more chlorine, the cleansing element, than does soy milk.

These factors are of extreme importance when we consider that many cases of insanity, neurasthenia, abnormal sex propensities and other disturbances of the nervous system are due chiefly to the unbalanced proportion of these elements in the food. The deficiency of chlorine in soy milk has a very important bearing on the flow and function of gastric juice in the stomach and may result in a deficiency of hydrochloric acid. It may also have a tendency to disturb the composition and activity of the blood serum which is largely composed of sodium and chlorine. Furthermore, these elements in soy milk are no longer organic when the soy material or the milk have been subjected to excessive heat.

In the final analysis, if the child cannot or does not want to drink milk, we can get the most nourishing food by feeding it fresh raw vegetable juices in a sufficient variety to supply its body with all the mineral and chemical elements, vitamins, hormones, calories and amino acids it needs. If the juices are properly made, fresh, from good quality fresh vegetables, the child cannot help but grow a strong, healthy, vital, energetic body strongly resistant to sickness and disease. As the infant grows, the juices may be supplemented with, but not supplanted by, finely grated vegetables and fruits, raw. Cooked and canned foods, cereals, grain and flour foods cannot build bodies resistant to sickness and disease. In the very nature of things and course of events, the body will develop means and ways in the shape of fevers, skin eruptions and ailments to rid itself of the waste matter resulting from the complete lack of life in such foods.

CREAM, and other FATS

While milk is a concentrated protein, cream is a fat purely and simply, and its digestion is entirely different. While of course it still is somewhat mucus-forming, it is nevertheless a fairly good fat, provided it is used in limited quantities. Cream should not be pasteurized. Animal fats are decidedly acid-forming, and when boiled or fried are likely to cause liver and gall bladder, as well as pancreas, disturbances. The best fats are avocado, olives and cold pressed olive oil.

CHEESE

The stronger the cheese, the greater is its acid-forming effect on the body, and the more mucus-forming it is. Cottage cheese (preferably the home-made kind) is probably the least mucus-forming, while the seasoned Swiss cheese, the kind that is made in huge round pieces about 3 feet across, and 8 or 10 inches thick, with large holes all through it, is the next best.

FROZEN FOODS

While heat, in cooking or processing, destroys the life element in vegetables, fruits, nuts and other food, quick freezing does not.

Quick freezing foods that are fresh and tree ripened maintain the life principle in suspension without in any way damaging or destroying the nourishing value of the food.

It is necessary, however, when un-freezing or defrosting such foods, to bear in mind that once their temperature is raised to the point where life in the atoms composing them becomes active, they are likely to spoil much quicker than in the case of fresh vegetables and fruits from the garden or from the market. The safe temperature to keep such foods after unfreezing them is about 34° to 38° F., provided they have not been warmed up to room temperature for more than 10 or 15 minutes.

Quick freezing has a tremendous advantage over other methods of keeping foods, as they can be kept frozen for many months without loss or deterioration if the quick freezing temperature is both fast and low enough to thoroughly freeze them. Another desirable feature is the tree or sun ripening of the vegetables and fruits which would make them a perishable product if so marketed without being quick frozen.

Many fruits are sweetened with sugar, and vegetables salted, when quick frozen commercially. It is well to watch for this condition when buying them, as sugar causes fruits to lose their nourishing value and gives an acid reaction in the body, while salt as an inorganic chemical tends to interfere with the organic processes of digestion.

PROTEIN

Protein is composed of Amino Acids. Amino acids are chains of atoms which, when combined, act, not only as building blocks for the building or construction of protein, but also have certain active functions which they perform, so long as there is life in the atoms composing such protein.

In other words, amino acids are not only the building blocks making up the protein, but, comparing them to an office or any other building, figuratively speaking, they represent all the activities that go on in such buildings.

In a building we have brick and mortar, lumber, hardware, etc., but we also have elevator service, hot and cold water, air circulating systems, sewage, lights, telephones, etc.

So in the protein of a live man or animal, the amino acids are the means of such a vast field of activities that no physical function is possible without them in live, vital, organic form.

The importance of VITALITY in the atoms composing the amino acids can best be appreciated by realizing that within 6 minutes after life leaves the body in death, all the atoms in the body cease to be live, organic atoms, and their function and activity consequently comes to a stop. So long as life is present in the body, the live atoms therein have the vital spark of life which enables them to carry on their work.

Atoms are not like animals whose life is apparent and perceived in active animation. Nevertheless, the vital life principle either is, or it is not present in an atom. If it is present, then the atom is a live organism capable of furnishing vital force and energy. If life is not present in it then the atom is inorganic and as such belongs to the mineral kingdom.

Nothing in Nature ever stands still. Things either progress, advance and develop, or they degenerate and disintegrate.

The mineral kingdom contains all the atoms composing this world, in inorganic form. Each of these atoms, while in the mineral kingdom state, has certain definite rates of vibration, but no life-principle is present. Their progress and development, we might say, is in reverse. As inorganic element compounds, they cannot develop constructively of their own account. They do however disintegrate, and when disintegrated they are collected by vegetation and by this means alone do they become instilled with the life-principle. It is only by means of this plant development that atoms can possibly become impregnated with life.

The very purpose of the creation of the Vegetable Kingdom was, and is, to give life to atoms, of converting mineral inorganic atoms into vital live organisms. When the life of vegetation is destroyed by heat, the atoms composing such vegetation automatically revert to the mineral kingdom state, as we cannot have life and death in anything at one and the same time.

To analyse some of the activities in which the amino acids are involved, we find that they are essential in the formation and growth of the blood, the normal operation of the glands, the healthy condition of the skin, of the hair, of the cartilage of the joints, the normal activities of the liver, and innumerable other functions which are regulated by the activity of one or more of the various amino acids, individually and collectively.

The protein composing the flesh of animals, fish and fowl, was built up in the respective bodies from the live, organic atoms in the raw food they were nourished with. Such flesh, of course, is a complete protein. Before the body can digest such protein, however, it must break it down not only into the original amino acids, but also into the original atoms in order that it may build up its own protein from these original atoms and primary amino acids.

It would be an insult to the intelligence of any normal individual to try to convince him that a dead horse can be ridden as efficiently as one that is living. Yet we find that the majority of people, including those who really should know better, still insist that the human body needs meat as an essential part of diet. In the first place the meat is poisoned when the animal is slaughtered, because of the poisons flowing into the animal's blood stream from the Adrenal glands through the terrified fear of the killing. In the second place such meat is a dead product deteriorating every second after the death of the animal. In addition, the meat and amino acids are still further destroyed by the heat in cooking.

Nevertheless, because of the habit of eating devitalized foods and existing in spite of this, it is difficult to convince people generally that the atoms in our food must be live, organic atoms if we hope or expect to build for ourselves a vital body free from sickness and disease. The lifeless, inorganic atoms in cooked and processed foods, by their very nature cause the degeneration and disintegration of the body.

Just as life is dynamic, magnetic, organic, so is death static, non-magnetic, inorganic. It takes life to beget life, and this applies to the atoms in our food. When the atoms in amino acids are live, organic atoms, they can function efficiently. When they are destroyed by the killing of the animal and the cooking of the food, the vital factors involving the atoms in the functions of the amino acids are lost.

All vegetables and fruits contain the necessary atoms from which amino acids are formed in the system. The human body cannot utilize for constructive purposes flesh products of any kind in the form of "complete proteins," but it can gather from the fresh vegetables and their juices, when these are fresh and properly made, the finest atoms from which to construct its own vital amino acids and protein.

The eating of meat, or any flesh products or extracts, in the very nature of things results in the accumulation of excessive amounts of acid, the most damaging of which is uric acid which the muscles absorb like a sponge absorbs water. As soon as the accumulation of this uric acid has reached the saturation point, it crystalizes, and the uric acid crystals form which are so painful in rheumatism, neuritis, sciatica, etc.

Animals build larger, huskier and healthier bodies from the amino acids obtained from vegetation, than man does by eating meat.

If more proof were needed to refute the farcical claims in favor of meat eating, we could look around for carnivorous animals suitable as beasts of burden— and find none, because they lack both power and endurance. Herbivorous animals, however, from the horse, the oxen to the elephant all have phenomenal strength and endurance obtained from eating raw vegetation.

WHAT ARE AMINO ACIDS? They are compound elements composed of carbon, hydrogen, oxygen and nitrogen atoms grouped in certain patterns and in certain definite proportions. Two of them, however, contain atoms of sulphur while two others contain atoms of iodine, in addition to these.

To give a non-technical description of amino acids, we could use the forms, patterns and colors of the petals of roses as a word picture. As these determine the various variety of roses, so these groups of atoms determine the type and variety of amino acids. The amino acids, in turn, group into patterns which form the different kinds of flesh protein.

The following are the principal amino acids, their composition, and their most important functions, activities and attributes:

1. Alanine: Composed of carbon 40%, hydrogen 8%, oxygen 36%, nitrogen 16%. Its molecular weight is about 89. It is a component of calcium pantothenate (one of the vitamin class) involved in the healthy condition of the skin, particularly that of the scalp, and of the hair. It is also a factor in the balance and healthy operation of the adrenal glands.

> The following raw foods contain alanine: Alfalfa, raw unsalted almonds, avocados, olives, cream, carrots, celery, dandelion, lettuce, cucumbers, turnips, green peppers, spinach, watercress, apples, apricots, grapes, oranges, strawberries, tomatoes.

2. Arginine: Composed of carbon 41½%, hydrogen 8%, oxygen 18½%, nitrogen 32%. Molecular weight, about 174. Involved in the contracting functions of the muscles; it is an important constituent of the cartilage, the tissue from which bones are formed by the natural process of calcification. It is essential in the structure and function of the reproductive organs. It helps to control the degeneration of body-cells, thus safeguarding the tissues from the formation of ulcers and cancer.

The following foods contain arginine: Alfalfa and other green vegetables, carrots, beets, cucumbers, celery, lettuce, leeks, radishes, raw potatoes, parsnips, turnips.

3. Aspartic Acid: Composed of carbon 36%, hydrogen 5½%, oxygen 48%, nitrogen 10½%. Molecular weight about 133. Helps to retard the destruction of bone and teeth, and protects the diffusion of calcium from the blood to the tissues. Involved in the functions of the lungs and respiratory channels and in the activities of the heart and of the blood vessels.

The following foods are sources of aspartic acid: Lemons, grapefruit, unsalted almonds, apples, apricots, carrot, celery, cucumber, parsley, pineapple, radishes, spinach, tomatoes, turnip tops, watercress and watermelon.

4. Cystine: Composed of carbon 30%, hydrogen 5%, oxygen 26½%, nitrogen 11½%, sulphur 27%. Molecular weight 240. One of the essential constituents of hair. Important element in the formation of red blood corpuscles. Active in the maintenance of health in the tissues and in resistance to poisons and infections. Involved in the functions of the mammary glands, particularly during lactation.

The following foods are sources of cystine: Alfalfa, carrots, beets, cabbage, cauliflower, chives, onions, garlic, kale, horseradish, radishes, Brussels sprouts, apples, currants, pineapple, raspberries, Brazil nuts, hazel nuts, filberts.

5. Glutamic Acid: Composed of carbon 41%, hydrogen 6%, oxygen 43½%, nitrogen 9½%, Molecular weight 147. Constitutes one-fifth of the components of the insulin molecule. Involved in the secretion of the digestive juices in the system and in the formation of glycogen. Essential in the action of amylolytic enzymes in changing glycogen into energy sugar through the liver. Its function is strongly disinfecting. It is a factor in the prevention of anemia, and in inhibiting or retarding the destruction of the functions of Vitamin C.

The following foods supply elements needed for glutamic acid: String beans and Brussels sprouts (raw), carrots, cabbage, celery, beet tops, turnip tops, dandelion, parsley, lettuce, spinach, papaya.

6.
Glycine: Composed of carbon 32%, hydrogen 7%, oxygen 42½%, nitrogen 18½%. Molecular weight 75. Involved in the formation of cartilage, and fibers of the muscles. It exercises a controlling influence on the excess generation of sex hormones.

The following foods are good sources of glycine: Carrots, dandelion, turnips, celery, parsley, spinach. Almonds (fresh, unsalted), alfalfa, okra, garlic, raw potatoes. Figs, oranges, lemons, huckleberries, raspberries, pomegranate, watermelon.

7.
Histidine: Composed of carbon 46%, hydrogen 6%, oxygen 21%, nitrogen 27%. Molecular weight 155. Active in the function of the liver in the formation of glycogen. Involved in the control of pathogenic mucus in the system. An important component of the hemoglobin of the blood and of the motile generative element of the semen which serves to impregnate the ovum at conception. It is therefore closely involved in pregnancy complications, such as abortion, premature and still births, sterility, etc.

The following foods are good sources of histidine: Horseradish, radishes, carrots, beets, celery, cucumbers, endive (chicory), leeks, garlic, onions, dandelions, turnip tops, alfalfa, spinach, sorrel, apples, pineapple, pomegranate, ripe and green papaya.

8.
Hydroxy-
glutamic Acid: Composed of carbon 37%, hydrogen 5%, oxygen 49%, nitrogen 9%. Molecular weight 163. Very similar in its functions to those of glutamic acid, with greater emphasis on its control over the generation of gastric juices in the system.

The following foods are good sources of supply: Carrots, celery, parsley, lettuce, spinach, tomatoes, grapes, huckleberries, raspberries, plums.

9.
Hydroxy-
proline: Composed of carbon 46%, hydrogen 7%, oxygen 36½%, nitrogen 10½%. Molecular weight 131. Involved in the activities of the liver and gall bladder, particularly in the emulsifying of fats and in counteracting their rancidity. Also involved in the formation of hematin and globulin in the red corpuscles of the blood.

The following foods are good sources of supply: Carrots, beets, lettuce, dandelions, turnips, cucumbers, almonds (unsalted), coconut, avocado, olives, apricots, cherries, Brazil nuts, figs, raisins, grapes (particularly Concords), oranges, pineapple.

10. Iodogorgoic Acid: Composed of carbon 25%, hydrogen 2%, oxygen 11%, nitrogen 3%, iodine 59%. Molecular weight 433. Involved in the functions of all the glands in the body, but particularly those of the thyroid, pituitary, adrenals, and lymph glands. (See the ENDOCRINE GLANDS CHART, by N. W. Walker, D.Sc., for the participating function of the glands, and the necessary vegetable juices to nourish them.)

The following foods contain iodogorgoic acid elements: Dulse, kelp, sea lettuce, carrots, celery, lettuce, spinach, tomatoes, pineapple.

11. Isoleucine: Composed of carbon 55%, hydrogen 10%, oxygen 24%, nitrogen, 11%. Molecular weight 131. Involved in the regulation of the thymus gland during childhood and adolescence, and the pituitary and spleen during adolescence and maturity, particularly in relation to growth and the regeneration of body tissues. Important factor in the regeneration of hemoglobin (red blood corpuscles). Helps the regulation of the general metabolism.

The following foods contain isoleucine elements: All nuts, except peanuts, cashews and chestnuts. Avocado, olives, ripe papaya, coconut, sunflower seeds, swiss cheese.

12. Leucine: Its composition and molecular weight are exactly like those of isoleucine. The difference is in the chain combination of the atoms which cause the leucine amino to rotate the plane of polarization to the left (levorotatory) while those of the isoleucine cause it to rotate to the right (dextrorotatory). As a result, leucine has a counter-balancing influence on the functions of isoleucine aminos.

The foods containing leucine elements are the same as those containing isoleucine elements.

13. Lysine: Composed of carbon 49%, hydrogen 10%, oxygen 22%, nitrogen 19%. Molecular weight 146. Involved in the functions of the liver and gall bladder, particularly in the metabolism of fats. Essential in the regulation and group participation of the pineal gland, the mammary glands, corpus luteum, oophoron and ovaries (female organs). Active in the prevention of degeneration of body cells and tissues.

Foods needed to supply lysine: Carrots, beets, cucumbers, celery, parsley, spinach, dandelion, turnip tops, green and ripe papaya, alfalfa, soy bean shoots (young, about 6 inches long), apples, apricots, pears, grapes.

14. Methionine: Composed of carbon 40%, hydrogen 7½%, oxygen 21½%, nitrogen 9%, sulphur 22%. Molecular weight 149. An important constituent of the hemoglobin of the blood, of the tissues and of the serum in the system. Involved in the functions of the spleen, the pancreas and the lymph glands.

Foods supplying methionine elements are: Brussels sprouts, cabbage, cauliflower (raw), sorrel, kale, horseradish, chives, garlic, watercress, pineapple, apples, Brazil nuts and filberts.

15. Norleucine: Another one of the leucine group, with composition and molecular weight like that of isoleucine (which see). Also known as glyco leucine. It is levorotatory, and helps to balance the functions and activities of the leucine group.

16. Phenylalanine: Composed of carbon 65½%, hydrogen 7%, oxygen 19%, nitrogen 8½%. Molecular weight 165. Involved in the processes of eliminating waste matter—both food waste and the used up cells and tissues in the body. Involved in the functions of the kidneys and bladder. Loses most of its efficacy in the presence of alcohol in the system.

Foods supplying the necessary elements in this connection, are: Carrot, beet, cucumber, spinach, parsley, tomatoes, pineapple, apples.

17. Proline: Composed of carbon 52%, hydrogen 8%, oxygen 28%, nitrogen 12%. Molecular weight 115. Involved in the activities of the white blood corpuscles or leucocytes. Also concerned in regulating the emulsifying of fats.

The following foods supply proline elements: Carrots, beets, lettuce, dandelions, turnips, cucumber, unsalted almonds, coconut, avocado, olives, apricots, cherries, Brazil nuts, figs, raisins, grapes, oranges, pineapple.

18. Serine: Composed of carbon 34%, hydrogen 7%, oxygen 46%, nitrogen 13%. Molecular weight 105. Involved in the cleansing of tissues in the system, particularly those concerned with the mucous membrane, the lungs and the bronchial tubes. Inefficient in the presence of nicotine (tobacco smoke).

The following foods contain serine elements: Horseradish, radishes, leeks, garlic, onions, carrots, beets, celery, cucumber, parsley, spinach, cabbage, alfalfa, papaya, apples, pineapple.

19.
Threonine:
Composed of carbon 48%, hydrogen 9%, oxygen 24%, nitrogen 19%. Molecular weight 142. Active in the exchange of amino acid atoms in the body, establishing the balance between their chain structure and their respective functions.
Food elements in: Ripe papaya, carrots, alfalfa, and other green leafy vegetables.

20.
Thyroxine:
Composed of carbon 23%, hydrogen 1½%, oxygen 8%, nitrogen 2%, iodine 65½%. Molecular weight 777. Involved in the activities of the thyroid, pituitary, adrenals and orchic glands, helping to regulate the general metabolism and speed of reactions, both voluntary and involuntary.
Foods containing thyroxine elements are: Dulse, kelp, sea lettuce, carrots, celery, lettuce, spinach, turnips, tomatoes, pineapple.

21.
Tryptophane:
Composed of carbon 65%, hydrogen 6%, oxygen 15%, nitrogen 14%. Molecular weight 204. Basic substance in the generation of cells and tissues in the body, from the primary sex cells to the completed tissues. Involved in the generation and functions of the gastric and pancreatic juices. Active in the efficiency of the optic system.
Foods necessary to maintain tryptophane equilibrium: Carrots, beets, celery, endive, dandelions, fennel, string beans (raw), Brussels sprouts (raw), chives, spinach, alfalfa, turnips.

22.
Tyrosine:
Composed of carbon 59½%, hydrogen 6%, oxygen 26½%, nitrogen 8%. Molecular weight 181. Essential in the generation of red and white blood corpuscles. Involved in the formation and development of body cells and tissues. Active in the functions of the adrenal, pituitary and thyroid glands. Active ingredient in the pigment cells of the hair.
Foods containing tyrosine elements: Alfalfa, carrots, beets, cucumbers, lettuce, dandelions, parsnips, asparagus tips (raw), leeks, parsley, green peppers, spinach, watercress, almonds (raw, unsalted), Swiss cheese, strawberries, apricots, cherries, apples, watermelon, figs.

23.
Valine:
Composed of carbon 51%, hydrogen 9½%, oxygen 27½%, nitrogen 12%. Molecular weight 117. Involved in the functions of the corpus luteum, mammary glands and ovaries, and their corresponding gland-group participation. See ENDOCRINE GLANDS CHART
Foods containing valine elements: Carrots, turnips, dandelions, almonds (raw, unsalted) lettuce, parsnips, squash (raw), celery, beets, parsley, okra, tomatoes, apples, pomegranate.

To clarify the chain combination of atoms in the various amino acids, it will suffice to give as examples those of the Leucine group:

LEUCINE: $(CH_3)_2CHCH_2CH(NH_2)COOH$.

(Empirical formula: $C_6H_{13}O_2N$)

ISOLEUCINE: $CH_3CH_2CH(CH_3)CH(NH_2)COOH$.

(Empirical formula: $C_6H_{13}O_2N$)

NORLEUCINE: $CH_3(CH_2)_3CH(NH_2)COOH$.

(Empirical formula: $C_6H_{13}O_2N$)

While these three amino acids have the same empirical atom formula, the manner in which these atoms combine changes the properties, activities and functions of each one.

When we consider the vast ramifications of these combinations of atoms and the work they have to perform, we can readily appreciate the value of LIFE in each atom. We can also appreciate the reason why it is so much more simple for the body to build its own complete live, efficient protein, than for it to disentangle the dead, lifeless atoms in the cooked flesh of animals.

It is a strange paradox that a whole community of civilized people will rise up in arms against an animal which has injured or killed a human being, yet it will flock in a festive mood to hunt and kill a helpless and defenseless bird or animal, then eat its lifeless remains. Worse still, it will nurse, nourish and protect from sickness and danger domesticated birds and animals, only to kill them, cook them and eat them with enjoyment!

The eating of meat is purely and simply a matter of personal taste, preference and judgment. It is very definitely not a matter of supplying the body with necessary protein.

Summarizing the meat situation, we find from practical experience that meat protein is both unnecessary for, and harmful to the human body. Heavy muscular work can be done better and with less fatigue when, as a habit, meat is entirely eliminated from the diet, and the necessary proteins are obtained from a variety of fresh raw vegetables and fresh vegetable juices which, extracted by means of a triturator and hydraulic press, contain all the elements which the body can use to build up its own protein.

Esthetically and morally, the killing of animals, birds and fish, cooking the flesh and eating the meat is not what Nature intended as nourishment for the human body. The life in such animals is placed there by the same Supreme Creator who placed a similar life within us. It is not our right, function or scope to deprive any animal of its natural life, any more than it is to deprive a human being of his life. In the matter of vibrations, the killing of animals, whether for sport or as a business, lowers the human vibrations several octaves. Eating their flesh lowers them still further, and automatically brings these down to the level of the vibrations of the animals. For example, the lower passions, alcoholic tendencies, nicotine habits and the general evanescence of inhibitions is definitely apparent in relation to the amount of meat consumed. Conversely, as meat disappears from the diet, better health, better and cleaner habits, greater understanding, more energy, vigor and vitality and a broader intellect are the natural sequence.

Physiologically, the eating of meat increases the acidity of the body. In the processes of digestion and the breaking down of the meat into its original amino acids, a vast amount of uric acid is generated in the body. If the body could eliminate this immediately, it might do only little harm. But what actually happens is that the muscles absorb enormous amounts of this uric acid, and in the course of time they are saturated with it. Eventually this acid forms into crystals with sharp needle-like points which cause the pain and discomfort known as rheumatism, neuritis, sciatica, nephritis (Bright's disease) or some diseases of the liver.

In the course of our researches we have made thousands of analyses of urine and without exception found that the urea present in the urine of meat eaters was only one-tenth to one-fifth of what should be eliminated, indicating that the muscles were absorbing from 5 to 10 times what the body should eliminate through the kidneys.

If for no other reason, we would refrain from eating meat or meat products because of our desire to avoid the aches and ailments resulting sooner or later from the accumulation of uric acid in the system.

RAW SALADS

Almost any combination of raw vegetables and fruits is compatible in salads. If the particular vegetables or fruits mentioned in the following recipes cannot be obtained in your locality use any others which may be available.

Regulate the amount of each ingredient according to individual taste and capacity. For an average salad one or two tablespoonfuls of each of the grated or chopped ingredients indicated will suffice. By using fruits and vegetables obtainable locally and using your own initiative and ingenuity, surprisingly delightful salads will result.

Use the following recipes simply as models, in the beginning, and learn therefrom how to prepare and combine the ingredients. Then dispense with the recipes and you will soon be surprised to find how simply you can concoct original and enjoyable salads.

If any dressing is desired, Health mayonnaise as described under "Salad Dressings", or cottage cheese or honey, or both, will be found delicious in that respect. Salad dressings containing vinegar, spices or preservatives are injurious to the system.

The general purpose here is to indicate how these several types of salads can be used either alone, or combined.

When trying out original ideas in salads it is a good plan, in order to avoid monotony, to use not more than two or three of the green vegetables, and include something sweet in the salad.

Onions are a very healthy addition to salad, but they should never be finely grated. When finely grated, the ethers in the onion may predominate in flavor and affect the entire salad. It is best to slice them or to chop them up not too finely.

Summer squash is another vegetable which it is best not to grate finely if used as a salad ingredient, but to cut it into small diced cubes. However, finely grated squash is a tasty addition to grated apples, as in raw apple sauce, with the addition of some honey for sweetening. The squash should be fresh and tender.

If lettuce or other vegetables suitable for garnishing are not available the salads can be very attractively arranged in soup dishes or plates, using nuts, and dried or fresh fruits to decorate the top.

After studying and preparing the following recipes one should be able to travel a new road of delightful salad discoveries.

HOW TO PREPARE THE VARIOUS VEGETABLES AND FRUITS

The proportions given in these salads are representative of the average amount for one serving.

Carrots
Beets
Turnips
Squash
White Radishes
Potatoes, etc.

When a recipe calls for these to be grated, 2 to 4 tablespoonfuls of each is plenty for one ingredient per salad. Grating can be done very well with an Acme Grater or similar utensil. When shredding is called for, then use a Schnitzler, Griscer or similar utensil, or just a plain shredder. (See page 51.) When diced or sliced, the dimensions should be as small as possible.

Leafy Vegetables

When chopped use a knife or chopper and cut as finely as possible. They may equally well be passed through a shredder or grater, and about 1 to 4 tablespoonfuls of each vegetable is ample per portion, according to the number of vegetables in the combination.

Cauliflower—raw

This should be cut into thin slices or it may be chopped finely—about 1 tablespoonful per salad.

Asparagus—raw

Can be chopped finely—use the tips and only as much of the stem as is not too fibrous. Use about 1 tablespoonful per helping.

Peppers

Can be grated, chopped or sliced. Use a b o u t 1 tablespoonful if grated or chopped, or about 4 rings if sliced.

Watercress

Use about 6 to 10 stalks with the leaves on them, per portion.

Avocados

Peel these, then cut into half slices and lay radially on the salad. Usually 6 to 10 slices suffice.

Broccoli

Use same as asparagus.

SALAD COMBINATIONS

NOTE: Salads 1 through 70 are 1 serving.

No. 1

Carrots, 2 tablespoonfuls	—finely grated
Lettuce, 2 tablespoonfuls	—finely chopped
Tomato, ½ medium sized	—divided into small segments
Celery, 2 tablespoonfuls	—finely chopped
Persimmon, ⅔ medium sized	—peeled and divided into segments
Raisins, 2 tablespoonfuls	—Thompson seedless preferably
Red Cabbage, 2 tablespoonfuls	—finely chopped
Banana, ½ large one	—diced
Dates, 2 large or 3 small	—cut into small segments
Radishes, 5 small	—finely sliced
Apple, 1 large	—shredded (preferably Delicious)
Avocado, ½ medium sized	—peeled and sliced lengthwise

For garnish—1 date, chopped walnuts, maraschino cherry, watercress.

Arrange each in layer beginning with carrots, one on top of the other up to and including the banana. Place radishes around the side of dish, grated apple in the center, avocado slices around sides, one date quartered placed cross-like in the center, nuts sprinkled over top and maraschino cherry in center. Garnish around edge with watercress.

No. 2

Celery, 2 tablespoonfuls	—finely chopped
Carrot, 2 tablespoonfuls	—finely grated
Lettuce, 2 tablespoonfuls	
Onion, 1 tablespoonful	—finely chopped and mixed together
Tomato, ½ medium sized	
Red Cabbage, 2 tablespoonfuls	—finely chopped
Banana Squash, 1 tablesp'nful —finely grated (on Acme)	
Apple, 1 Delicious, shredded	
Fig, 1 large, cut in segments	Mix all together.
Honey, 2 teaspoonfuls	
Walnuts, 2 tablespoonfuls, chopped	
Avocado, ½ medium sized	—peeled and sliced lengthwise
Radishes, 5 small	—use whole
Olives, stuffed	
Parsley	

(continued on next page)

Arrange in several layers as follows—celery, then carrot, the mixture of lettuce, onion and tomato, red cabbage, then in the center the banana squash, apple, etc., mixture. Place avocado slices and radishes around sides, stuffed olives in center and garnish with parsley.

No. 3

Asparagus (raw), 1 or 2 stalks, fresh and crisp	
String beans (raw), 6 fresh and crisp	Finely chopped
Lettuce, 1/4 head, fresh and crisp	—Coarsely chopped
Parsley, 2 tablespoonfuls	—Finely minced
Carrot, 1 small	—Finely grated (on Acme)
Cottage Cheese, Farmer's style preferably, 2 ounces	
Pecan and Walnut halves, 4 or 5	
Peach, 1/2 large fresh	
Avocado, 1/2 medium sized	—Peeled and cut lengthwise
Lettuce leaves	

Mix all of above together in a bowl, except the peach, avocado, some of the nut meats and a little of the cottage cheese. Arrange crisp leaves of lettuce on dinner plate and place this mixture on plate in the form of a mould. Cover this entire mould with thin slices of peach and garnish with thin slices of the avocado. Place the remaining cottage cheese in the center and sprinkle with finely chopped nut meats.

No. 4

Lettuce, 1/4 head crisp and fresh	—Coarsely chopped
Celery, 2 or 3 stalks	—Finely chopped
Cucumber, 1/2 large (do not peel)	—Finely grated*
Parsley, 1 tablespoonful	—Finely minced
Onions, 3 or 4 small green	—Finely chopped
Asparagus (raw) 2 or 3 stalks, fresh and crisp	—Finely chopped
Cauliflower, 2 teaspoonfuls	—Finely grated
Beets, 2 medium sized, fresh, young	—Finely grated
Peas, fresh tender green, 1 or 2 tablespoonfuls	—Use whole
Avocado, 1/2 medium sized	
Lettuce leaves	

Arrange crisp leaves of lettuce on dinner plate and place the above vegetables in layers, each in the rotation given, sprinkling the whole green peas over the top of the beets and garnishing with the strips of avocado. (*If the cucumber is grated, including the peeling, on an Acme Grater, this makes the peeling very fine and easy to masticate and also brings out the juice of the cucumber giving moisture and flavor to the salad.)

No. 5

Lettuce, ¼ head crisp, fresh	
Celery, 1 or 2 stalks	—Chopped fine
Irish Potato (raw with skin on) ½ small	—Diced very small
Carrot, 1 medium sized	—Finely grated
Onion, Sweet Spanish, ½ large size	—Finely chopped
Green Pepper, 1 teaspoonful	—Finely chopped
Tomatoes, 2 small or 1 large ripe	—Peeled and cut in thin slices
Cottage Cheese, preferably Farmer Style, 2 ounces	
Avocado, ½ medium sized	—Peeled, cut lengthwise
Lettuce leaves or endive	

Arrange all the chopped and grated vegetables in mound on crisp leaves of lettuce or endive, cover with slices of tomato, garnish with strips of avocado and top with mound of cottage cheese sprinkled with paprika.

No. 6

Lettuce, ½ head solid, crisp	—Chopped
Avocado, ½ large	—Peeled and sliced lengthwise
Pineapple, 4 slices (preferably fresh or canned unsweetened)	
Cottage Cheese, 3 ounces (preferably Farmer Style)	
Parsley, 1 tablespoonful	—Finely minced
Red Pepper, sweet, few strips	
Endive or lettuce leaves	

Arrange chopped lettuce on bed of endive or lettuce leaves and cover with layer of cottage cheese. Arrange strips* of avocado across the center of the dish and place strips of pineapple on either side. Sprinkle very finely chopped parsley over all this and garnish with thin strips of sweet red pepper. (*The avocado may be sliced with a wire egg slicer.)

No. 7

Lettuce, ½ head solid, crisp	—Chopped fine
Carrots, 1 or 2 large crisp	—Finely grated (on Acme)
Raisins, seedless, ¼ cupful	
Cottage Cheese, 3 ounces	
Honey	

Arrange chopped lettuce on plate or dish, cover with grated carrot and one-half of raisins mixed together. Sprinkle with 1 teaspoonful or more of honey, cover with cottage cheese and garnish with the balance of the raisins.

No. 8

Cabbage, ½ cupful, fresh crisp	—Finely chopped
Celery, ½ cupful	—Diced
Parsley, 1 tablespoonful	—Finely minced
Spinach, 3 or 4 leaves	—Finely chopped
Carrot, 1 large	—Finely grated
Honey, 1 tablespoonful	
Cottage Cheese, 2 or 3 ounces	

Apples, 1 large grated—or—grated unsweetened Pineapple
Parsley, red sweet pepper or radishes for garnish

Arrange layers of cabbage, celery and spinach on dinner plate. Cover this with the grated carrots and sprinkle as evenly as possible with 1 tablespoonful of honey, cover with cottage cheese and top with grated apple or pineapple. Garnish with sprigs of parsley and strips of red sweet pepper or radish rings.

No. 9

String Beans (raw and fresh), 6 or 7	—Grated fine
Asparagus (raw and fresh), 4 or 5 stalks	—Chopped fine
Cucumbers, ½ large (including skin)	—Grated fine
Green Pepper, 1 teaspoonful	—Grated
Celery, 2 or 3 stalks, crisp	—Grated or finely chopped
Carrots, 1 or 2 large crisp	—Finely grated
Pecan meats, ¼ cupful	—Finely chopped
Grapes, Thompson Seedless, ½ cupful	—Cut in halves or quarters
Peaches, 1 large fresh ripe	—Slice thinly lengthwise

Mix all the above ingredients together in bowl, except peaches, nuts and a few grapes. Arrange mixture on crisp lettuce leaves, cover with sliced peaches and garnish with nuts and grapes cut in halves. Honey may be added if desired.

No. 10

Lettuce, ¼ head	—Chopped
Asparagus (raw fresh) 2 or 3 stalks	—Finely chopped
Green Onions, 4 or 5—or—Sweet Spanish Onion, ½ large	—Finely chopped
Green Pepper, 1 tablespoonful	—Finely chopped
Celery, 2 or 3 stalks crisp	—Finely chopped
Tomatoes, 2 medium sized firm ripe	—Peeled and sliced
Cottage Cheese, 2 ounces	

Mix these all together except the tomatoes and a little of the cottage cheese. Arrange in mound on crisp leaves of lettuce and cover with thin slices of tomato. Top with cottage cheese and a dash of paprika.

No. 11

Irish Potato (raw with skin), ½ medium sized	—Finely grated
Carrot, 1 small	—Finely grated
Celery, 2 or 3 stalks crisp	—Finely chopped
Parsley, 1 tablespoonful	—Finely minced
Green Pepper, 1 teaspoonful	—Finely grated
Apples, 1 large juicy	—Grated
Beets, 2 medium sized young	—Grated finely
Nuts, ¼ cupful (pecans or walnuts)	—Finely chopped

Mix these all together except the apples and beets and a few of the nuts. Arrange this mixture on crisp leaves of lettuce, cover with layer of grated apple and top with layer of grated beets sprinkled with the chopped nuts.

No. 12

Red Cabbage, ½ cupful	—Finely chopped
Asparagus, 3 or 4 stalks	—Finely cut
Green Onions, 3 or 4	—Finely chopped
Celery, 3 or 4 stalks fresh crisp	—Grated or finely chopped
String beans (raw fresh), 4 or 5	—Grated
Tomatoes, 1 or 2 large firm ripe	—Peeled and ½ sliced and ½ diced
Cucumber, ½ medium sized	—Run fork lengthwise of cucumber pressing hard enough to break skin; slice thinly
Green Pepper, 1 teaspoonful	—Finely grated
Cottage Cheese, 2 ounces	
Paprika and Marjoram	

Mix cabbage, asparagus, onions, celery, string beans, one tomato diced, the green pepper and most of the cottage cheese, together in a bowl. Sprinkle lightly with Marjoram (one of the herbs which can be bought at grocery stores in powdered form). Arrange in mound on plate garnished with lettuce leaves or endive and cover with sliced tomato, top with remaining cottage cheese and arrange the cucumber slices around outer edge of salad. Add a dash of paprika to the cottage cheese and cucumber slices.

No. 13

Red Cabbage, 1 tablespoonful	—Finely chopped
Lettuce, ¼ head crisp	—Finely chopped
Celery, 2 tablespoonfuls	—Finely cut

(continued on next page)

Salad 13 - continued

Parsley, 1 teaspoonful	—Finely minced
Green Pepper, ¼ teaspoonful	—Finely grated
Cottage Cheese, 1 teaspoonful (Farmer's style)	—made into two balls
Avocado, ½ large	—Peeled and cut lengthwise

Ripe Olives

Celery stuffed with avocado paste to which has been added ground almonds

Beets, 1 or 2 tablespoonfuls, young tender—Finely grated

Mix cabbage, lettuce, celery, parsley and green pepper together and form in mould. Place in center of plate garnished with crisp lettuce leaves or endive, top with grated beet and surround with slices of avocado, arranging the two cottage cheese balls, sprinkled with paprika, on either side of the mound. Serve with ripe olives, and crisp celery stuffed with avocado paste and almonds (made by mashing ripe avocado and whipping to smooth creamy consistency, then mixing in finely chopped or ground almonds).

No. 14

Lettuce, ½ head crisp fresh	—Finely chopped
Spinach, 6 or 8 leaves	—Finely chopped
Parsley, 1 tablespoonful	—Finely minced
Green Onions, 6 or 8	—Finely chopped
Cucumber, ½ large fresh crisp unpeeled	—Thinly sliced
Watercress	

Garnish plates with lettuce leaves or endive. Mix spinach, parsley, onions and watercress together and sprinkle over this. Cover with sliced cucumbers and a dash of paprika.

No. 15

Green Onions, 3 or 4	—Finely chopped
Romaine Lettuce, 3 or 4 fresh crisp leaves	—Finely chopped
Parsley, 1 tablespoonful	—Finely minced
Radishes, 3 or 4 fresh crisp	–Finely cut
Celery, 3 or 4 stalks	—Finely chopped
Asparagus, 3 or 4 stalks (raw)	—Finely cut
Peas, fresh tender green (raw) ¼ cupful	—Whole
Cucumber, ½ medium sized incl. peel	—Grated
Tomatoes, 1 medium sized firm red, or 2 small	—Peeled and cut in wedges

Mix these all together, except the tomatoes, and arrange in mound on leaves of lettuce or endive. Surround with wedges of tomato. Swiss cheese is delicious served with this.

No. 16
(One Serving)

Lettuce, ½ small firm crisp head	—Finely chopped
Celery, 2 or 3 stalks	—Finely chopped
Parsley, 2 tablespoonfuls	—Finely minced
Tomatoes, 2 medium sized firm ripe	—Peeled and sliced
Avocado, ½ large ripe	—Peeled and cut lengthwise

Garnish plate with endive and cover this with the chopped lettuce, celery and parsley; then with sliced tomatoes and avocado arranged alternately.

No. 17

Lettuce, ¼ head crisp	—Finely chopped
String Beans (raw) fresh green, 4 or 5	—Finely chopped
Cucumber, ½ large with skin	—Grated
Watercress, 3 or 4 sprigs	—Finely minced
Green Pepper, 1 teaspoonful	—Finely grated
Tomatoes, 1 large ripe firm	—Peeled and sliced
Avocado, ½ medium sized	—Peeled and sliced lengthwise

Cottage Cheese, 2 ounces

Mix all the chopped and grated vegetables together and arrange in mound on crisp lettuce. Cover with sliced tomatoes and arrange slices of avocado around edge. Top with the cottage cheese.

No. 18

Tomatoes, 1 very large smooth, red, firm	—Cut off the top, scoop out the center and slightly scallop the top edge.
Celery, 3 or 4 stalks crisp	—Finely chopped
Green Onions, 3 or 4	—Finely chopped
Cucumber, ½ medium sized with peel	—Grated
Cottage Cheese, 2 ounces	
Ripe Olives, 4 large	
Green Pepper, sweet	

After scalloping edge of tomato cut down through corners to form flower-like petals and spread open on plate garnished with endive. Fill the center with the following — the center part removed from tomato, chopped celery, green onions and cucumber, with enough cottage cheese to hold the mixture together. Top with the balance of the cottage cheese and garnish with very thin strips of sweet green pepper and the ripe olives.

No. 19

Apples, 1 very large or 2 small	—Peeled, cored and sliced in rings less than ¼ inch thick, dipping in lemon juice immediately.

(continued on next page)

Parsley, 1 tablespoonful	—Finely chopped
Celery, 3 or 4 stalks crisp	—Finely minced
Avocado, ½ large ripe	

Arrange the chopped celery on beds of endive or crisp lettuce leaves. Peel the avocado and cut in thin rings around the seed, placing one on each apple ring. Arrange these decoratively over the bed of chopped celery and sprinkle with the minced parsley. Strips of Swiss cheese may be served with this.

No. 20

Cabbage, 1 cup crisp	—Finely chopped
Celery, 2 or 3 stalks	—Finely chopped
Ripe Olives, 5 or 6 large	—Cut into small pieces
Radishes, red, small, crisp 4 or 5	—Cut in small pieces
Sour Cream	

Mix these all together, saving out a few radishes for garnishing. Mix sufficient sour cream to suit the individual taste. If it tastes flat add a little vegetable salt. Serve on romaine lettuce bed covering top with very thin slices of radish.

No. 21

Lettuce, ¼ head, crisp	—Chopped
Celery, 3 or 4 stalks	—Finely chopped
Persimmons, 1 large or 2 small, very ripe	—Peel and cut in sections
Cottage Cheese, 2 or 3 ounces	
Date, ½ large for garnish	

Arrange lettuce and celery on endive, cover with sections of persimmon and top with the cottage cheese with half of date in center.

No. 22

Lettuce, ½ small crisp head	—Finely chopped
Celery, 3 stalks	—Finely chopped
Prunes, fresh or dried, *½ cupful	—Cut from seeds into small pieces
Apples, ripe juicy, 1 large	—Finely grated
Cream, sweet whipped, ½ cupful (preferably raw)	Sweeten with honey
Walnuts	

Mix together the celery, lettuce, prunes and apples and add enough whipped cream, sweetened with honey, to make the right consistency. Serve on crisp beds of lettuce topped with the balance of the whipped cream and finely cut walnut meats. *If dried prunes are used, soak in tepid water overnight or until soft. Do not cook.

No. 23
(One Serving)

Tomatoes, 1 or 2 large firm ripe	—Peeled and cut in wedge-like sections
Avocado, ½ large ripe or 1 small	—Peeled and cut lengthwise
Cottage Cheese, 2 or 3 ounces	
Endive	

Arrange endive on dinner plate and place tomato sections alternately with slices of avocado around outer edge. Mould cottage cheese in center with a dash of paprika.

No. 24
(One Serving)

Pineapple, Unsweetened Tidbits, ½ cupful	
Pear, ½ medium sized	—Grated
Apple, 1 small (Delicious preferably)	—Grated
Cabbage, ½ cupful crisp	—Finely chopped
Pecans	
Cream, sweet whipped, ½ cupful (preferably raw)	—Sweetened with honey

Mix pineapple, pear, apple and cabbage lightly with two forks and add about half of the whipped cream. Arrange on bed of crisp lettuce and garnish with balance of the whipped cream and pecans.

No. 25

Cabbage, ½ cupful crisp	—Finely chopped
Parsley, 1 tablespoonful	—Finely minced
Celery, 2 stalks crisp	—Finely chopped
Carrots, 1 large	—Finely chopped
Honey, 1 tablespoonful	
Cottage cheese, 2 ounces	
Apples, 1 small or medium sized (Delicious)	—Grated
Avocado, ½ small	—Peeled and cut lengthwise

Arrange above in order given on bed of lettuce on dinner plate, using avocado around edge for garnish. A sprig of parsley or watercress may be placed in center.

No. 26

Turnips, sweet young white, 1 medium sized	—Grated
Red cabbage, crisp, ½ cupful	—Finely chopped
Celery, 1 or 2 stalks, crisp	—Finely chopped
Parsley, 1 tablespoonful	—Finely minced
Romaine lettuce, ½ small head	—Finely chopped
Avocado, ½ medium sized	—Peeled and cut lengthwise

(continued on next page)

Salad 26 - continued

Mix these all together with a little Health Mayonnaise, tossing lightly with two forks, and serve on boats made of Romaine lettuce leaves, garnished with sliced avocado, sprinkled with paprika.

No. 27

No. 1	Cabbage, ½ cupful crisp	—Finely chopped
	Green Pepper, 1 teaspoonful	—Finely chopped
	Celery, 1 or 2 stalks, crisp	—Finely chopped
	Sour Cream Dressing	
No. 2	Celery, 4 or 5 stalks, crisp	—Finely chopped
	Carrot, 1 small	—Finely grated
	Health Mayonnaise	
No. 3	Celery, 1 or 2 stalks, crisp	—Finely chopped
	Beet, 1 medium sized young tender	—Finely grated
	Lettuce, ½ head, small crisp	—Finely chopped

For Garnish: 3 or 4 small red radishes, ¼ avocado and green pepper.

Mix the three above combinations separately in the order in which the ingredients are listed, using the amount of dressing desired in each, and place in moulds. Arrange endive on a large dinner plate and unmould these three combinations in center, leaving at least 1-inch space between them, so they will not be jumbled together. Garnish No. 1 with thin slices of crisp red radishes; No. 2 with spears of avocado and No. 3 with thin strips of green pepper and one stuffed olive. Serve stuffed olives, Swiss cheese and celery hearts.

No. 28

Cabbage, ⅓ cupful crisp	—Finely chopped
Celery, 3 or 4 stalks	—Finely chopped
Lettuce, ¼ small crisp head	—Finely chopped
Carrot, 1 medium sized	—Finely grated
Green Pepper, 1 teaspoonful	—Finely chopped
Cottage Cheese, 2 ounces	
Marjoram, a dash	
Sour cream dressing	

For Garnish: ¼ avocado cut in strips, sweet red pepper strips

Mix vegetables together, with sour cream to suit taste, tossing lightly with two forks. Arrange this mixture in mould in center of crisp lettuce or endive with a dash of Marjoram. Top with cottage cheese and garnish with avocado and sweet red pepper strips. Serve celery stuffed with cream cheese and chopped pecans.

Bananas, 1 or 2 very ripe — —Diced
Lettuce, ¼ small crisp head — —Finely chopped
Celery, 2 or 3 stalks crisp — —Finely chopped
Raisins, seedless, 1 tablespoonful
Pear, ½ ripe firm — —Diced
Cream, sweet whipped, ½ cupful
  (preferably raw) — —Sweetened with honey
Nuts (pecans or walnuts) 2 tablespoonfuls—Finely chopped

Mix all these with part of the whipped cream and some of the nuts, and arrange in mould on crisp lettuce or endive. Top with balance of whipped cream and nuts.

No. 30

Apples, 1 or 2 ripe juicy Jonathans — —Grated finely
Spinach, 5 or 6 leaves, crisp fresh — —Finely chopped
Celery, 3 or 4 stalks — —Finely chopped
Red Cabbage, ⅓ cupful — —Finely chopped
Parsley, 1 tablespoonful — —Finely minced

Mix half of grated apple with chopped vegetables, except parsley. Arrange in center of bed of crisp lettuce and cover with remaining apple and minced parsley. With this may be served thin slices of Swiss cheese, either imported or domestic type.

No. 31

Grapefruit, 1 large ripe sweet — —Peel and remove membrane from sections
Avocado, ½ large ripe but firm — —Peel and cut lengthwise
Lettuce, ½ small solid crisp head — —Finely chopped
Celery, 3 or 4 stalks — —Finely chopped
Cottage Cheese, 2 or 3 ounces
Pecans, 1 tablespoonful

Garnish dinner plate with crisp lettuce or endive and make complete wheel around outer edge using grapefruit sections and thin slices of avocado alternately. Mix together the chopped lettuce and celery, half of the cottage cheese and all but one of the pecan halves, finely chopped. Arrange this in center of plate and top with balance of the cottage cheese and a pecan half. Add a dash of paprika.

No. 32

Spinach, ½ large fresh bunch — —Very finely chopped
Avocado, ½ large ripe — —Peeled and mashed until fluffy
Celery, 2 or 3 stalks — —Finely chopped
Onion, sweet Spanish, ¼ medium sized — —Finely chopped
Tomatoes, 2 medium sized ripe firm red—Scoop out centers
Ripe olives and green sweet pepper for garnish

(Continued on next page)

Salad 32 - continued

Mix together the spinach, avocado, celery and onion and fill tomato shells. Place on dinner plate on bed of endive and garnish top with thin strips of green sweet pepper and place ripe olive in center of each stuffed tomato. This may be served with celery hearts, ripe olives and strips of Swiss cheese.

No. 33

Spinach, ½ large fresh bunch	—Very finely chopped
Apples, 1 or 2 small juicy	—Finely grated
Persimmons, 1 large or 2 small, very ripe	—Peel and cut in sections
Celery, 2 or 3 stalks	—Finely chopped
Cottage Cheese, 1 or 2 tablespoonfuls	
Avocado, ½ small	—Peeled and cut lengthwise

Mix spinach, apples, persimmons and celery together and serve on bed of lettuce topped with cottage cheese and garnished with strips of avocado and a dash of paprika.

No. 34

Lettuce, ½ small crisp solid head	—Finely chopped
Cabbage, ¼ cupful crisp	—Finely chopped
Irish Potato (raw), ¼ medium sized	—Finely grated
Almonds, ¼ cupful	—Grated or ground
Green Pepper, sweet, 1 teaspoonful	—Finely chopped
Cottage Cheese, 1 or 2 ounces	
Pecan halves, 6 or 8	
Avocado, ½ small	—Peeled and cut lengthwise

Dash of Marjoram

Mix together the lettuce, cabbage, potato, green pepper, Marjoram and almonds and arrange on bed of crisp lettuce or endive. Cover outer edge of mound with slices of avocado and pecan halves. Top with cottage cheese and dash of paprika.

No. 35

Carrots, 1 medium sized	—Finely grated
Spinach, ½ bunch fresh crisp	—Finely chopped
Lettuce, ¼ head firm crisp	—Finely chopped
Parsley, 1 tablespoonful	—Finely minced
Cottage Cheese, 2 or 3 ounces	
Apple, 1 large Delicious	—Grated
Avocado, ¼ medium sized	—Peeled and cut lengthwise
Dates, 4 or 5	—Finely chopped
Honey, 1 teaspoonful	

Mix together in bowl the carrots, spinach, lettuce and parsley and to this add about 1 tablespoonful of cottage cheese to which enough cream has been added to make it the consistency of salad dressing. Place this mixture on bed of crisp lettuce on dinner plate, sprinkle with honey and cover with layer of chopped dates. Add layer of grated apple and top with balance of cottage cheese and strips of avocado with a dash of paprika.

No. 36

Cabbage, ⅓ cupful, crisp	—Finely chopped
Celery, 3 or 4 stalks, fresh crisp	—Finely chopped
Parsley, 1 tablespoonful	—Finely minced
Honey, 1 teaspoonful	
Apple, 1 large Delicious	—Grated
Banana, ½ large ripe	—Thinly sliced
Persimmons, 1 medium or 2 small, ripe	—Peel and cut in sections
Cottage Cheese, 1 or 2 ounces	

Garnish dinner plate with endive and arrange the above in layers in the order given except persimmons and cottage cheese. Arrange sections of persimmons around outer edge of layers and top with cottage cheese, with sprig of parsley or watercress in center.

No. 37

Spinach, ½ bunch fresh crisp	—Finely chopped
Carrots, 1 large	—Finely grated
Lettuce, ¼ small crisp head	—Finely chopped
Celery, 2 or 3 stalks	—Finely chopped
Avocado, ⅓ large	—Peel, mash and beat until light and fluffy
Cottage Cheese, 2 or 3 ounces	
Apple, 1 medium sized juicy	—Grated
Parsley, 1 tablespoonful	—Chopped
Honey, 1 teaspoonful	

Mix together the spinach, lettuce, celery and mashed avocado and arrange a layer of this on dinner plate garnished with crisp leaves of lettuce or endive. Cover this with layer of grated carrots, sprinkle with honey and add layer of cottage cheese, then grated apple, and garnish with chopped parsley.

No. 38

Cabbage, ⅓ cupful, crisp	—Finely chopped
Dates, 5 or 6	—Finely chopped
Parsley, 1 tablespoonful	—Finely minced
Lettuce, ¼ head solid crisp	—Finely chopped
Watercress, several sprigs	—Finely minced
Honey, 1 teaspoonful	
Apple, 1 large or medium sized Delicious	—Grated
Cottage Cheese, 2 or 3 ounces	
Avocado, ¼ large	—Peeled and cut lengthwise

(continued on next page)

. 69

Salad 38 - continued

Garnish dinner plate with endive or crisp leaves of lettuce and cover with layer of cabbage, then dates and parsley, lettuce and watercress and sprinkle with honey. Cover this with layer of apple, then cottage cheese. Arrange thin slices of avocado around outer edge of mound, place sprig of parsley in center. Add a dash of paprika.

No. 39

Lettuce, ¼ head solid crisp	—Finely chopped
Celery, 2 or 3 stalks	—Finely chopped
Carrot, 1 medium sized	—Grated
Figs, *Black Mission, 3 or 4	—Finely cut
Watercress, several sprigs	—Finely chopped
Cottage Cheese, 2 or 3 ounces	
Apple, 1 large or medium sized juicy	—Finely grated
Honey, 1 teaspoonful	

Arrange Romaine lettuce on dinner plate and add layers of lettuce, celery, carrots, figs and watercress. Sprinkle with honey and cover with cottage cheese, topping with grated apple and sprig of watercress. *If dried figs are used, soak until soft in tepid water; do not cook.

No. 40

Celery, 3 or 4 stalks	—Finely chopped
Lettuce, ¼ small crisp head	—Finely chopped
Parsley, 1 tablespoonful	—Finely minced
Beets, 2 small or medium, fresh tender	—Finely grated
Apple, 1 large Delicious	—Grated
Cottage Cheese, 2 or 3 ounces	
Honey, 1 teaspoonful	

Arrange layer of celery, lettuce and parsley on bed of crisp endive and sprinkle with honey. Cover with layer of grated beets, then apple and top with cottage cheese and a dash of paprika with a sprig of parsley in center.

No. 41

Winter pears, 2 large juicy	—Cut in cubes
Lettuce, ½ head crisp firm	—Cut in medium sized chunks
Dates, 5 or 6	—Finely cut
Cream, sweet whipped, ½ cupful (preferably raw)	—Sweetened with honey

Mix enough of whipped cream with pears, lettuce and dates to suit the individual taste and serve in boats made of Romaine lettuce. Top with the balance of whipped cream and one-half date.

Carrot, 2 tablespoonfuls	—Finely grated
Spinach, 2 tablespoonfuls	—Finely chopped
Banana, ½ medium sized ripe	—Diced
Raisins, 2 tablespoonfuls	
Red Cabbage, 2 tablespoonfuls	—Finely chopped
Lettuce, 2 tablespoonfuls, crisp fresh	—Finely chopped
Green pepper, 2 tablespoonfuls	—Finely chopped
Persimmon, ½ large	—Peeled and divided in segments
Apple, 1 medium sized Delicious	—Grated
Avocado, ⅓ medium sized, ripe	—Peeled and cut lengthwise
Parsley, several sprigs	
Almonds, raw, 8 or 10	—Whole or chopped

Place on crisp lettuce leaves a layer of grated carrot, then spinach, and spread each of the other ingredients one on top of the other in the order mentioned. The persimmon segments may be arranged around the center of mixture and the slices of avocado radially around this, using parsley and whole or chopped almonds for garnish.

No. 43

Cabbage, 2 tablespoonfuls	—Finely chopped
Spinach, 2 tablespoonfuls	—Finely chopped
Celery, 2 tablespoonfuls	—Finely chopped
Broccoli, 1 tablespoonful	—Finely chopped
Peas, raw, fresh, tender, green, 2 tablespoonfuls	
Cottage Cheese, 2 ounces	
Honey	
Apple, 1 medium sized Delicious	—Finely grated
Green Pepper, 1 ring	
Radish, 1 medium or large red	

Arrange above in a large soup dish, layer by layer in order given. Sprinkle the cottage cheese with honey before adding the grated apple. Save out two teaspoonfuls of cottage cheese for garnish. Lay green pepper ring in center of apple layer, place cottage cheese in center and top with the radish.

No. 44

Lettuce, 2 tablespoonfuls	—Finely chopped
Celery, 2 tablespoonfuls	—Finely chopped
Spinach, 2 tablespoonfuls	—Finely chopped
Green Pepper, 1 tablespoonful	—Finely chopped
Peas, raw, fresh, tender, green, 2 tablespoonfuls	
Cauliflower, raw, 1 large flower	

(continued on next page)

Salad 44 - continued
Radishes, red, 3 made into roses

—This is done by thoroly cleaning radishes, cut off top, take one slice from tail end and with paring knife gently peel the red skin back like petals from the tail end.

Avocado, ½ medium sized
Apple, 1 medium sized Delicious
Cottage Cheese, 2 ounces
Honey

Arrange in large soup dish by layers the lettuce, celery, spinach, green pepper and peas. Dot with cottage cheese and sprinkle with honey. Save about one teaspoonful of cottage cheese for garnish. Add the apple finely grated. Place the cauliflower in center. Divide the cottage cheese into three dabs equidistant around cauliflower and place a radish rose in center of each dab. Arrange thick slices of avocado around outer edge.

No. 45

Cabbage, 2 tablespoonfuls	—Finely chopped
Lettuce, 2 tablespoonfuls	—Finely chopped
Celery, 2 tablespoonfuls	—Finely chopped
Broccoli, 1 tablespoonful	—Finely chopped
Spinach, 1 tablespoonful	—Finely chopped

Green Pepper, 1 ring
Apple, 1 medium sized, sweet and ripe
Cottage Cheese, 2 ounces
Radish, red, 1 rose—(see salad No. 44)
Honey

Arrange finely chopped vegetables in layers on plate or in large soup dish, top with half the cottage cheese, sprinkle with honey, cover with the apple finely grated. Arrange balance of cottage cheese in mound in center and on top of this place green pepper ring with the radish rose in center.

No. 46

Beet, red and sweet, raw, 2 tablespoonfuls	—Very finely grated on Acme-type grater
Celery, 2 tablespoonfuls	—Diced
Cabbage, 2 tablespoonfuls	—Finely chopped
Apple, 1 medium sized sweet	—Diced
Whipped Cream, 2 tablespoonfuls	
Walnuts, 2 tablespoonfuls	—Finely cut or sliced

Honey

Mix together the grated beet, celery, cabbage, apple and half the whipped cream (which has been sweetened to taste with honey). Arrange in soup dish and top with remaining whipped cream and sprinkle the chopped or sliced walnuts over it all.

Cabbage, 2 tablespoonfuls	—Finely chopped
Celery, 2 tablespoonfuls	—Finely chopped
Broccoli, 1 tablespoonful	—Finely chopped
Cauliflower, 1 tablespoonful	—Finely chopped
Spinach, 1 tablespoonful	—Finely chopped
Cottage Cheese, 2 ounces	
Apple, 1 medium sized sweet	—Finely grated
Green Pepper, 1 ring	
Red Pepper, sweet, 2 rings	
Honey	

Arrange the chopped vegetables in soup dish in layers in order given above. Top with half of cottage cheese, sprinkle with honey, add layer of grated apple and place remaining cottage cheese in center topped with green pepper ring. Cut the two red pepper rings in half, arrange three of the halves around edge of salad and dice the fourth half on top of cottage cheese inside green pepper ring.

No. 48

Cabbage, 2 tablespoonfuls	—Finely chopped
Celery, 2 tablespoonfuls	—Finely chopped
Cauliflower, 1 tablespoonful	—Finely chopped
Carrot, 1 tablespoonful	—Finely grated
Broccoli, 1 tablespoonful	—Finely chopped
Spinach, 1 tablespoonful	—Finely chopped
Green Pepper, 3 rings	
Cottage Cheese, 2 ounces	
Apple, 1 medium sized sweet	—Grated
Honey	
Radishes, 3 red	
Olive, 1 ripe	

Arrange the chopped and grated vegetables in layers in soup dish in order given. Top with half the cottage cheese, sprinkle with honey, cover with layer finely grated apple. Arrange green pepper rings around outer edge of salad and place a radish in center of each. Put remaining cottage cheese in middle of salad and top with the ripe olive.

No. 49

Cabbage, 2 tablespoonfuls	—Finely chopped
Spinach, 2 tablespoonfuls	—Finely chopped
Celery, 2 tablespoonfuls	—Finely chopped
Summer Squash, 1 medium sized green scalloped, raw	—Diced
Green Pepper, 2 rings	
Cottage Cheese, 2 ounces	
Tomatoes, 2 medium sized or 1 large	—Sliced

The chopped vegetables can be arranged in layers,

(continued on next page)

add the diced summer squash, half the cottage cheese and top with the sliced tomatoes. Garnish with the balance of cottage cheese and green pepper rings.

No. 50

Cabbage, 2 tablespoonfuls	—Finely chopped
Spinach, New Zealand (or regular)	
1 tablespoonful	—Finely chopped
Celery, 2 tablespoonfuls	—Finely chopped
Radish, 1 red	
Summer Squash, Zucchini,	
2 tablespoonfuls, raw	—Diced
Cucumber, ½ medium sized	—Diced
Onion, Sweet Spanish, 1 tablespoonful	—Finely chopped
Green Pepper, 1 ring	
Tomatoes, 2 medium sized or 1 large	
firm ripe	—Sliced
Cottage Cheese, 2 ounces	

Chopped and diced vegetables can be arranged in layers in soup plate or on regular dinner plate. Dot with half the cottage cheese, cover with sliced tomatoes with balance of cottage cheese in center topped with green pepper ring and radish in center.

No. 51

Cabbage, 2 tablespoonfuls	—Finely chopped
Spinach, 1 tablespoonful	—Finely chopped
Celery, 2 tablespoonfuls	—Finely chopped
Onion, sweet, 1 tablespoonful	—Finely chopped
Summer Squash, green scallop, 1 medium	
sized, raw	—Diced
Green Pepper, 1 ring	
Avocado, ½ medium sized ripe, firm	—Sliced lengthwise
Cottage Cheese, 2 ounces	
Tomatoes, 2 medium sized ripe, firm	

Arrange layers of chopped and diced vegetables, top with half the cottage cheese then add the sliced tomatoes. Place slices of avocado around top of salad like flower petals, or spokes in a wheel. Place balance of cottage cheese in center and top with green pepper ring.

No. 52

Cabbage, 2 tablespoonfuls	—Finely chopped
Lettuce, 2 tablespoonfuls	—Finely chopped
String Beans, raw, fresh and crisp,	
1 tablespoonful	—Finely chopped
Celery, 2 tablespoonfuls	—Finely chopped
Spinach, 1 tablespoonful	—Finely chopped
Green Pepper, 1 ring	

(continued on next page)

Avocado, ½ medium firm ripe
Cottage Cheese, 2 ounces
Tomatoes, 2 medium sized firm ripe

Place layers of the chopped vegetables in order given in large soup dish. Dot with half the cottage cheese, cover with the sliced tomatoes. Dice the avocado in center of salad, top with remaining cottage cheese and dice the green pepper on top of the cottage cheese.

No. 53

Lettuce 1 tablespoonful	—Finely chopped
Cabbage 2 tablespoonfuls	—Finely chopped
Celery 1 tablespoonful	—Finely chopped
Asparagus (raw) 1 stalk	—Finely chopped
Peas (raw) 1 tablespoonful	
Bell Pepper 3 rings	—2 rings finely chopped
Apple (Delicious) 1	—Acme grated
Avocado ½ ripe, medium sized	
Onions, Spring Green, 1 tablespoonful	—Finely chopped
Carrot 1 medium sized, 1 teaspoonful	—Acme grated
Vegetable Salt	
Honey	

Arrange the lettuce, cabbage, celery, asparagus, peas and the 2 rings of bell pepper finely chopped, in layers in order given, in a deep soup plate. Over this, spread the grated apple on which, or in which, add a little honey. Make a smooth, cream-like mixture of the avocado (by mashing and whipping it with a fork) in which the spring, or young, green onion, finely chopped, is thoroly mixed with one teaspoonful of honey (warm the honey so it flows easily) and add a little vegetable salt to taste. Spread this mix over the apple, covering the entire salad. Place the one ring of bell pepper on top, in the center, in the middle of which put one heaping teaspoonful of the finely grated carrot. In the center of the carrot place either a radish-rose, or an olive, or a sprig of parsley or the small leafy heart of a celery bunch, like a palm tree in the desert, for decoration.

No. 54

Bibb Lettuce, 2 tablespoonfuls coarsely cut	—Bibb Lettuce is very tender and delicious, not usually procurable in markets.
Celery, 2 tablespoonfuls	—Diced
Cucumber, ½ medium sized	—Diced
Green Pepper, 4 rings	
Radishes, red, 4 to 6 medium sized	—Diced

(continued on next page)

Avocado, ½ medium sized	—Sliced lengthwise
Cottage Cheese, 2 ounces	
Tomatoes, 2 medium sized firm ripe	—Sliced lengthwise in thick wedges

Arrange Bibb lettuce and diced vegetables in layers in order given. Dot with half the cottage cheese. Arrange lengthwise slices of the avocado and tomatoes alternately over top and place remainder of cottage cheese in center.

No. 55

Bibb Lettuce (if not available use any lettuce that is), 2 tablespoonfuls	—Coarsely cut
Green Pepper, 5 rings	—Finely chopped
Cabbage, 2 tablespoonfuls	—Finely chopped
Celery, 2 tablespoonfuls	—Finely chopped
Cucumber, ½ medium sized	—Diced
Peas, raw fresh green and tender, 1 tablespoonful	
Cottage Cheese, 2 ounces	
Tomatoes, 2 medium sized	—Sliced

Place lettuce and chopped and diced vegetables in layers in order given. Spread layer of half the cottage cheese over top, cover with the sliced tomatoes and form the remaining cottage cheese into an indented mound in center and place the fresh green peas in center of this mound.

No. 56

Bibb Lettuce, or other green leafy lettuce, 2 tablespoonfuls	—Coarsely cut
Spinach, 2 tablespoonfuls	—Finely chopped
Celery, 2 tablespoonfuls	—Diced
Cucumber, 1 medium sized	—Diced
Tomatoes, 2 medium sized or 1 large	
Avocado, ½ medium sized	

Mix lightly together with two forks the lettuce, spinach, celery, cucumber, and half the tomatoes which have been cut in wedges. Garnish with the remaining tomato and avocado.

No. 57

Bibb Lettuce, or other green leafy lettuce, choose uniform leaves, crisp and fresh	
Cucumber, 1 medium sized	—Diced
Celery, 2 tablespoonfuls	—Diced
Green lima beans, raw, fresh, and young, 2 tablespoonfuls	
Spinach, 2 tablespoonfuls	—Finely chopped
Avocado, ½ medium sized	—Thinly sliced
Tomatoes, 2 medium sized or 1 large	
Cottage Cheese, 1 teaspoonful	

(continued on next page)

Arrange lettuce leaves around outer edge of dinner plate. In center place layers of the diced cucumber and celery, lima beans and spinach. Cover this with slices of avocado. Cover with thin slices of tomato and place cottage cheese in center.

No. 58

Cucumber, 1 medium sized	—Diced
Celery, 2 tablespoonfuls	—Diced
Tomatoes, 2 medium sized firm ripe	—Diced
Avocado, ½ medium sized	—Diced
Swiss Cheese, 2 ounces	—Diced

Toss lightly together with two forks the above ingredients and serve either plain or on a bed of crisp lettuce leaves.

No. 59

Lettuce, 2 tablespoonfuls	—Finely chopped
Cabbage, 2 tablespoonfuls	—Finely chopped
Spinach, 1 tablespoonful	—Finely chopped
Celery, 2 tablespoonfuls	—Finely chopped
Summer Squash, dark green Zucchini, 1 tablespoonful	—Finely chopped
String Beans, raw fresh and tender, 1 tablespoonful	—Finely chopped
Green Pepper, 1 ring	
Avocado, ½ medium sized	—Thinly sliced
Tomatoes, 2 medium sized	—Thinly sliced
Cottage Cheese, 1 ounce	

Arrange finely chopped vegetables in soup dish or on dinner plate, in order given above. Cover with sliced avocado, then sliced tomatoes and top with the cottage cheese.

No. 60

Cabbage, 2 tablespoonfuls	—Finely chopped
Spinach, 1 tablespoonful	—Finely chopped
Celery, 2 tablespoonfuls	—Finely chopped
String Beans, 2 tablespoonfuls	—Finely chopped
Cucumber, ½ medium sized	—Diced
Green Pepper, 3 rings	
Avocado, ½ medium sized	—Thinly sliced
Tomatoes, 2 medium sized	—Thinly sliced
Cottage Cheese, 1 ounce	

Place the chopped and diced vegetables in layers in order given. Cover with thin slices of avocado, then add the sliced tomatoes. Place the three green pepper rings edge to edge on top. Make the cottage cheese into three balls and put one in center of each green pepper ring.

Lettuce, 2 tablespoonfuls	—Finely chopped
Cabbage, 2 tablespoonfuls	—Finely chopped
Celery, 2 tablespoonfuls	—Finely chopped
Spinach, 2 tablespoonfuls	—Finely chopped
Wax String Beans, raw, fresh, tender, 1 tablespoonful	—Finely chopped
Cucumber, ½ medium sized	—Diced
Cottage Cheese, 2 ounces	
Tomatoes, 2 medium sized or 1 large	

Arrange in layers the diced and chopped vegetables. Dot with half the cottage cheese, cover with the tomatoes thinly sliced and make a cross of the remaining cottage cheese in center.

No. 62

Lettuce, 2 tablespoonfuls	—Finely chopped
Radishes, red, 4 or 5	—Finely chopped
Celery, 2 tablespoonfuls	—Finely chopped
Spinach, 2 tablespoonfuls	—Finely chopped
Summer Squash, Zucchini, 1 tablespoonful	—Diced
Cucumber, ½ medium size	—Cut in slices about ⅛" thick
Green Pepper, 3 rings	—Diced
Tomatoes, 2 medium sized or 1 large	
Cottage Cheese, 2 ounces	

Place the chopped and diced vegetables, except the green pepper, in layers on dinner plate, dot with half the cottage cheese and cover with thinly sliced tomatoes. Mix the diced green pepper with the remaining cottage cheese and form into mound in center of salad. Arrange the slices of cucumber on plate around edge of salad.

No. 63

Celery, 2 tablespoonfuls	—Finely chopped
Lettuce, 2 tablespoonfuls	—Finely chopped
Spinach, 1 tablespoonful	—Finely chopped
Cabbage, 2 tablespoonfuls	—Finely chopped
Summer Squash, green scallop, 1 tablespoonful	—Diced
Green Pepper, 1 ring	
Whipped Cream, 2 tablespoonfuls	—Sweetened with honey
Fresh Peach, ½ large ripe, sweet	
Grapes, Thompson Seedless, ripe and sweet, 1 tablespoonful	
Figs, fresh and ripe, 4 or 5 large	

Toss together lightly with two forks the chopped and diced vegetables with one tablespoonful of the whipped cream. Place in large soup dish and cover with thin slices of peach. Peel the figs and arrange diagonal sections around outer edge of dish. Place remaining whipped cream in center and sprinkle with the grapes which have been carefully stemmed and washed. If this salad is not sweet enough sprinkle with honey.

No. 64

Celery, 2 tablespoonfuls	—Finely chopped
Lettuce, 2 tablespoonfuls	—Finely chopped
Spinach, 1 tablespoonful	—Finely chopped
Summer Squash, dark green Zucchini, 1 tablespoonful	—Diced
Green Pepper, 3 rings	
Avocado, ½ medium sized	
Fresh Peaches, ripe and sweet, 2 small or 1 large	
Fresh Figs, 4 or 5 large	—Peeled and diced
Walnuts, 2 tablespoonfuls	—Finely chopped
Honey	

Arrange in layers in large soup dish the chopped and diced vegetables, cover with thin slices of avocado. Add layer of thinly sliced peaches, sprinkle with honey. Place the three green pepper rings edge to edge in center of dish and fill each with the diced figs and sprinkle with the chopped walnuts.

No. 65

Cabbage, 2 tablespoonfuls	—Finely chopped
Lettuce, 2 tablespoonfuls	—Finely chopped
Celery, 2 tablespoonfuls	—Finely chopped
Spinach, 1 tablespoonful	—Finely chopped
Summer Squash, Zucchini, 1 tablespoonful	—Diced
Green Pepper, 1 ring	
Pear, fresh, 1 small or ½ large	
Fresh figs	
Cottage Cheese, 2 ounces	
Honey	

Arrange chopped and diced vegetables in large soup dish, in layers as given above. Dot with half the cottage cheese and sprinkle lightly with honey. Take very thin peeling off the pear and thinly slice over cottage cheese. Lay green pepper ring in center and fill with remaining cottage cheese. Peel figs and arrange in diagonal slices around edge of salad. Sprinkle lightly with honey.

No. 66

Cabbage, 2 tablespoonfuls	—Finely chopped
Celery, 2 tablespoonfuls	—Finely chopped
Lettuce, 2 tablespoonfuls	—Finely chopped
Summer Squash, green scallop, 1 tablespoonful	—Diced
Green Pepper, 2 rings	

(continued on next page)

Salad 66 - continued

Fresh Peaches, 2 small or 1 large ripe sweet
Fresh Figs, 4 or 5 large
Cottage Cheese, 2 ounces
Honey

Fill large soup dish with layers of chopped and diced vegetables, spread with half the cottage cheese and sprinkle lightly with honey. Cover with very thinly sliced fresh peaches. Peel and cut figs in wedges lengthwise and arrange in strip across dish from one edge to the opposite edge. Place a green pepper ring on either side of this. Form remaining cheese into two balls and place one in each green pepper ring. Sprinkle lightly with honey.

No. 67

Cabbage, 2 tablespoonfuls	—Finely chopped
Celery, 2 tablespoonfuls	—Finely chopped
Spinach, 1 tablespoonful	—Finely chopped
Green Pepper, 2 tablespoonfuls	—Finely chopped
Raisins, Thompson Seedless, soaked, 2 teaspoonfuls	
Cottage Cheese, 2 ounces	
Pear, fresh, 1 small or ½ large	
Peaches, 2 small or 1 large	
Honey and finely cut almonds	

Place chopped vegetables in layers, sprinkle with raisins, dot with half the cottage cheese and sprinkle with honey. Peel and slice the peaches lengthwise and arrange in layer around outer edge of dish. Dice the pear very finely and fill in the center. Top with the remaining cottage cheese and sprinkle with finely cut almonds. More honey can be added if not sweet enough to suit taste.

No. 68

Celery, 2 tablespoonfuls	—Finely chopped
Spinach, 1 tablespoonful	—Finely chopped
Cabbage, 2 tablespoonfuls	—Finely chopped
Green Pepper, 2 tablespoonfuls	—Finely chopped
Avocado, ½ medium sized	
Pear, fresh, 1 large	
Figs, fresh, 6 large	—Peeled and cut in lengthwise sections
Grapes, dark red sweet Tokays	—Cut 10 or 12 in halves, remove seeds
Honey	
Walnuts, 2 tablespoonfuls	—Finely chopped

Arrange in layers the chopped vegetables, sprinkle lightly with honey. Cover with layer sliced avocado and add layer thinly sliced pears. Place halved grapes

in center and surround with fig sections. Sprinkle
with honey and walnuts.

No. 69

Cabbage, 2 tablespoonfuls	—Finely chopped
Spinach, 2 tablespoonfuls	—Finely chopped
Celery, 2 tablespoonfuls	—Finely chopped
Summer Squash, green scallop, 1 tablespoonful	—Diced
Avocado, ½ medium sized	
Peaches, 2 small or 1 large sweet	
Grapes, sweet Malagas, 6 or 8 seeded	—Diced
Cottage Cheese, 2 ounces	
Honey	
Green Pepper, 1 ring	

On a dinner plate arrange layers of chopped and
diced vegetables, cover with half the cottage cheese
and sprinkle lightly with honey. Cover with very
thinly sliced peaches and sprinkle very lightly with
honey. Mix together the diced grapes and remaining
cottage cheese and form a mound in center topped with
green pepper ring. Place avocado sliced lengthwise
around outer edge of salad on edge of plate.

No. 70

Cucumber, ½ medium sized	—Diced
Celery, 2 tablespoonfuls	—Finely chopped
Summer Squash, Zucchini or green scallop, 2 tablespoonfuls	—Diced
Spinach, 2 tablespoonfuls	—Finely chopped
Parsley, 2 tablespoonfuls	—Finely chopped
Cabbage, 1 tablespoonful	—Finely chopped
Tomatoes, 2 medium sized	—Cut in small chunks
Green Pepper, 2 rings	
Olive Oil, 1 or 2 teaspoonfuls	
Green Ripe Olives, 3	

Toss together lightly with two forks all of the
vegetables and tomatoes, place in large soup dish and
sprinkle with the olive oil. Garnish with the three
green pepper rings placing an olive in the center of
each.

This is delicious served plain or with thin slices of
Swiss cheese.

MENUS

The juice of 1 whole lemon in 6 or 8 ounces of hot
water immediately upon arising—(no sweetening).
The general effect of this is to flush the liver and the
kidneys. (If cold water is used it will be more likely
to stimulate the peristaltic action of the intestines.)

(continued on next page)

In 15 to 30 minutes, drink a glass of fresh orange juice.

15 to 30 minutes later:

BREAKFAST

1 or 2, 8-ounce glasses of fresh raw vegetable juice, either carrot juice—as a general mental tonic, or raw potassium (carrot, celery, parsley and spinach) as a blood food (and also to clear the mind of the effects of "the morning after," if this is needed. Straight celery juice is also good for this), or carrot and spinach if the elimination is at all sluggish, or carrot, beet and cucumber juice as a food for the liver, gall bladder and kidneys.

For many people this juice breakfast will be sufficient. Others will want a little more food, in which case try the following:

No. 1

Bananas, 1 or 2 good ripe (no green on either end)—sliced.
Cream, sweet (preferably raw)
Honey, if sweetening desired
Carrot juice, fresh, 8-ounce glass
Note: If a heavier breakfast is desired, nuts (except peanuts), figs, dates, raisins, persimmons or cottage cheese may be added to the above, either separately or combined to suit the taste.

No. 2

Apples* 1 or 2 medium sized   —Grated or shredded
Cream, sweet (preferably raw)
Date sugar or honey for sweetening
Carrot and Spinach juice, fresh, 8-ounce glass.
*Many prefer Delicious apples; experiment with different kinds for a few mornings until you find the one best suited to your taste and digestion.
For a more substantial breakfast the above can be covered with 1 or 2 tablespoonfuls of cottage cheese and a few nuts (unsalted almonds, pecans or walnuts).

No. 3

Pears, 1 or 2, grated or shredded, may be used instead of the apples in No. 2 breakfast.
Carrot, Beet and Cucumber juice (combined, raw and fresh), 8-ounce glass.

No. 4

Pears, 1 or 2 medium sized, first layer—Grated or diced
Apple, 1 large Delicious, second layer—Grated

Date sugar or honey for sweetening, and cream if
   desired.
Nuts, 1 or 2 tablespoonfuls (any kind except peanuts)
Cottage Cheese, 1 or 2 tablespoonfuls
Carrot and Celery juice combined, fresh, 8-oz. glass.

No. 5

Peaches, apricots, berries and other fresh fruits, when
   in season, either all one kind or mixed.
Cream, sweet (preferably raw)
Honey for sweetening
Carrot juice, fresh, 8-ounce glass, or carrot and celery
   or straight celery juice. (These are the best juices
   with this type of breakfast.)

*Note: The addition of some figs and dates, whole or chopped,
adds variety to any of the above dishes.*

No. 6
Omelet

*(Sometimes a more substantial breakfast is wanted by one
accustomed to a large morning meal that sticks to the ribs. Then
we find eggs useful.)*

Egg yolks, 2 or 4 (no whites) ⎫ Beat together these
   according to size   ⎪ ingredients and place
Cream, sweet, 1 large table- ⎬ in heavy iron skillet
   spoonful to each 2 yolks   ⎪ which has been pre-
Vegetable salt   ⎭ viously heated and
in which a little butter has been allowed to melt. Cook
over a low flame until set and slightly brown under-
neath, then place skillet under medium high broiler
flame until delicately browned on top.

*This can be placed on a plate and used as a base making a
variety of dishes, for example: Cover with thin layer of grated
apple, or any one of the varieties or combinations of fruit outlined
in the preceding breakfast menus, or, place 2 or 3 tablespoonfuls of
cottage cheese on the omelet and top this with a layer of grated
apple or other fruit.*

Carrot juice, fresh, 8-ounce glass, or straight celery
   juice.
Celery 2 or 3 stalks, or some lettuce *(this is a good
addition to every breakfast).*

   Cereals are unnecessary and of no value whatsoever
either as nourishment or for energy, unless one is
anxious to increase the acid condition of the body.
   Prunes, while somewhat acid-forming, have a laxative effect which makes them a popular dish for breakfast. It is not necessary to cook prunes. It is best to
soak them for several hours or overnight in tepid water.

LUNCH

The best lunch to eat in the middle of the day, to avoid the fatigue which results from the indiscriminate eating of incompatible foods usually served in restaurants, etc., is the following:

No. 1

Vegetable juice, fresh and raw, 1 or 2 pints

Apples, 1 or 2 large, or pears, or bananas, ripe, or 1 or 2 lbs. of grapes, or any other fresh fruit in season in like quantity. One, two or more different fruits may be eaten during lunch.

No. 2

A more substantial lunch:

Cheese*, Swiss, 2 to 4 ounces

Apples, 1 or 2 large juicy

Vegetable juice, fresh and raw, 1 or 2 pints

Celery, several stalks, some spinach, lettuce, watercress or other green vegetable, raw.

*The American Swiss cheese (with holes in it), Wisconsin or similar good quality cut from the large round block, is as good as the imported. (The processed, in squares in packages, is somewhat more acid-forming.)

One week's trial of lunches chosen from these suggestions should prove to the most skeptical that sandwiches, doughnuts and the like are the cause of that let-down condition, that fatigue, which overtakes us in mid-afternoon. Peanuts are exceedingly acid-forming.

No. 3

Dates, raisins, figs and nuts, handful, separately or mixed.

Celery, 3 or 4 stalks, or some lettuce, spinach, parsley or other green vegetables.

Vegetable juice, fresh raw, 1 pint (straight celery, potassium or carrot)

Note: When a heavier meal is required in the middle of the day, then choose a suggestion from the Dinner Menus and use the Lunch Menu in the evening.

It is a good plan, whenever possible, to drink a pint or two of fresh vegetable juices between meals. One pint at least of fresh raw carrot juice in mid-afternoon, for example, works wonders, while in hot weather a pint of straight celery juice helps to keep the body temperature normal and so make the heat more bearable. The use of ordinary salt in drinking water in hot weather or at any other time has the tendency eventually towards hardening arteries.

DINNER

It is an excellent plan to start dinner with at least an 8-ounce glass of fresh raw vegetable juices. This is much more digestible than soup. Straight celery or carrot juice is one of the best juices to drink just before eating a meal.

For the next course, use any one of the salads outlined in the Salad section, particularly one of the more elaborate. A sufficient number of salads is given to permit of an untiring variety. It is seldom that more food is wanted after eating one of these. However, if dessert is desired fruit is best. Use any kind that seems most suitable with the salad served.

Think of the saving of labor in dishwashing!

RAW FOOD MENUS — DINNER

No. 1 — Salad No. 2
Carrot juice, fresh raw, 8-ounce glass
Fruit for dessert (if desired) for example: 2 or 3 sections of ripe peeled persimmon, ½ pear diced; top with 1 or 2 teaspoonfuls of whipped cream sweetened with honey, or serve plain with some grated almonds on top.

No. 2 — Salad No. 3
Celery juice straight, fresh raw, 8-ounce glass
Strawberries with honey and cream for dessert (if desired).

No. 3 — Salad No. 11
Carrot and Celery juice, fresh raw, 8-ounce glass
Peaches, fresh juicy, sprinkled with date sugar or honey (if desired).

No. 4 — Salad No. 15
Serve with Swiss cheese, 2 or 3 ounces to each serving.
Potassium Broth, fresh raw, 8-ounce glass.
Raspberries, red fresh, served plain or with honey and cream (if desired)

No. 5 — Salad No. 18
Carrots and Celery juice, fresh raw, 8-ounce glass.
Cherries, sweet ripe, served on stems or pitted and halved in sherbet dishes.

No. 6 — Salad No. 21
Carrot, Celery and Parsley juice, fresh raw, 8-oz. glass.
Grapes (if desired) large purple Tokay, 1 medium sized bunch.

No. 7 — Salad No. 27
Serve with Swiss cheese, 2 or 3 ounces to each serving, stuffed olives and celery hearts.
Apple and Pomegranate juice, fresh raw, 1 8-oz. glass.

Fresh pineapple strips sprinkled with honey and topped with whipped cream sweetened with honey, and grated or finely chopped almonds.

Note: This is a good "Guest" dinner as it is slightly more elaborate than some of the others.

Raw food dinners can always be dressed up and made very colorful and attractive by the addition of radishes, green onions, ripe or stuffed green olives, celery hearts, sliced cucumbers, sliced raw carrots or strips of raw carrot cut thin, lengthwise, sliced raw potatoes, Jerusalem artichokes, whole or sliced, green pepper rings, raw cauliflower hearts, nuts, dates, figs, etc., attractively arranged in odd dishes. Colored pottery dishes add much to the service of raw foods. Food that appeals to the eye as well as the taste will digest better, and therefore a little extra time devoted to making meals attractive is well spent.

A diet of all raw foods without an abundance of raw vegetable juices, is not sufficient, due to the inability of the body to handle the large volume of raw fiber in vegetables to obtain the necessary amount of the mineral elements.

Therefore raw foods are just as essential when drinking juices, as raw vegetable juices are when eating raw foods.

If difficulty is experienced in the body handling too much raw food in the beginning, then drink a correspondingly greater quantity of raw vegetable juices and eat plenty of raw fruits, as their fiber is more readily digested and is nearly as efficient.

We must remember that the body will need less food if it is raw than if it is cooked. The calories idea of arranging a meal by calory portions is nonsense. Raw foods contain all the calories and all the elements the body requires, particularly if supplemented with plenty of raw vegetable juices. It is not calories we need as nourishment. We need chemical elements, minerals and salts in organic live form, their vitamins and enzymes.

Overeating

To fill a stomach with more than it is intended to hold for digestive purposes, means stuffing it unduly. Overloading the stomach overtaxes all the functions of the body and shortens life.

After all, the normal capacity of the average stomach is equivalent to about one quart.

Overeating the right kind of foods, even in correct combinations, still overworks all the organs of the body.

Eat only sufficient food to be comfortable. Don't think that a stuffed stomach is well-fed. Better far a mite of hunger after a meal than indigestion.

Vegetarian-cooked holiday menus for those who feel they must have cooked food at this time. The combinations are compatible.

SUGGESTION FOR THANKSGIVING DINNER

Appetizer—Small glass fresh Apple and Celery juice

Celery Hearts   Green Ripe Olives   Radish Roses

VEGETARIAN NUT LOAF

Carrot Juice   Carrot and Celery Juice
Fresh Green Peas, buttered   Diced Buttered Beets
Cranberry Jelly
Green Salad
Fruit Delight with Whipped Cream

* * *

Vegetarian Nut Loaf

8 cups carrot pulp, grated on Acme-type grater (very fine)
1 cup fresh green Lima Beans (these can be purchased frozen)
2 large onions, finely chopped
10 egg yolks
2 tablespoonfuls finely chopped parsley
1 cup broken Cashew nuts
1 cup finely flaked almonds
6 tablespoonfuls melted butter
3 teaspoonfuls vegetable salt
2½ teaspoonfuls Sage
2 teaspoonfuls Thyme

Mix grated carrots and other vegetables together in large bowl. Squeeze some of the juice from the grated carrots into the egg yolks, add salt and spices and beat thoroly then mix with the vegetables. Add nuts and melted butter and mix very thoroly. Bake in greased pyrex loaf pan in moderate oven until done, about 1 hour. Serve on plates in slices just thick enough to hold together. This amount serves 12 people.

Note: Cook the peas and beets until they are barely tender with as little water as possible. Season with little vegetable salt and butter and serve immediately. Do not start to cook them until everything is nearly ready to serve and hover over them to make sure that they do not overcook in which case they will retain their bright color and flavor.

* * *

Green Salad

Mix together equal parts of chopped cabbage, spinach, celery, cucumber, green pepper and tomatoes. Sprinkle with olive oil and serve on crisp leaves of lettuce. Garnish with sprigs of parsley.

Fruit Delight

Finely diced pears, dates and chopped walnuts. Sweeten with honey and serve cold topped with whipped cream (also sweetened with honey).

Cranberry Jelly Made With Honey

4 cups washed cranberries (be sure to remove all soft ones or those with spots)

2 cups water

½ cup honey to each cup strained pulp

⅛ cup lemon juice to each 4 cups strained pulp

Cook until berries pop open and are tender. Rub through sieve or collander. Measure sieved pulp and add honey and lemon juice. Cook until it reaches the boiling point and boil hard for 7 minutes, stirring constantly. Remove from fire and pour into sterilized glasses in the usual way.

NOTE: Read on page 110 paragraph on Cranberries.

SUGGESTION FOR CHRISTMAS DINNER

Appetizer—Tomato juice served cold in small cups, to which has been added a bit of very finely grated onion and finely chopped green pepper and celery

Carrot Strips   Ripe Olives   Radishes

CARROT SOUFFLE

Apple Juice   Carrot and Celery Juice

Steamed Onions   Broccoli

Fresh Green Peas

Stuffed Celery Salad

Cinnamon Apple with Whipped Cream

* * *

Carrot Souffle

6 egg yolks

6 tablespoonfuls water

½ teaspoonful vegetable salt

2 cups triturated (or finely grated) raw carrot pulp

Thoroly beat the egg yolks, water and salt and fold in the carrot pulp with a fork. Pour in a greased pyrex baking dish, square or oblong, about 1½ or 2 inches deep, and bake in a hot oven 450° until done. When a silver knife dipped in cold water and inserted in the Souffle comes out clean it is done. Serve on plates in squares covered with steamed onions. Serves 8 people.

Steamed Onions

The onions can be steamed in their own juice and a bit of olive oil in a casserole dish in the oven while the Souffle is baking. Remove from oven just as soon as tender and sprinkle with yellow grated cheese and a little paprika and place under the broiler just long enough to melt the cheese. Allow 2 medium sized onions for each serving desired. They should be finely chopped before cooking.

* * *

Cook the peas and broccoli just long enough to break up the fibers, remove from fire, season with vegetable salt and butter and serve at once.

* * *

Stuffed Celery Salad

Clean and de-string celery. Prepare a small dish of finely chopped parsley and one of finely grated carrot. Mix honey with cottage cheese and fill center of tender crisp celery. Top with some grated carrot and sprinkle with parsley. Cut in strips about 2 inches long and arrange 4 or 5 on crisp lettuce leaves.

Cinnamon Apple With Whipped Cream

Finely grate sweet apples (Delicious are preferable) and season with honey and cinnamon. Serve in sherbet glasses topped with whipped cream sweetened with honey and finely chopped almonds.

Nut Dressing Supreme

3 cups finely cut celery
6 cups finely grated carrots
¾ cup finely cut onion and parsley
1 cup chopped walnuts
1½ teaspoonfuls of sage
1 cup broken pieces raw cashew nuts
Vegetable salt
Olive oil or butter

Prune Whip

Wash well and soak prunes in water until thoroughly soft. Drain, pit and put through food chopper, then through colander. Mix with the prune pulp one-third as much flaked pignolias and beat well together with a rotary beater. A little honey may be added if desired but prunes are usually sufficiently sweet. Top with whipped cream and a sprig of mint.

A perfectly good meal can be ruined by using—crackers or bread for stuffing—bread and butter, gravy made with flour —potatoes—cake or pie crust made with flour. By omitting from the meal all food containing flour, starch or sugar it will be entirely compatible and should not upset the digestion.

* * *

SALAD DRESSINGS*
Health Mayonnaise

2 egg yolks   1 teaspoonful honey
¼ teaspoonful vegetable salt   1 teaspoonful lemon juice
1 pint vegetable oil

Mix all ingredients, except oil, in bowl and beat together. Slowly add the oil a drop or two at a time until the mixture is the right consistency. If used on fruit salad a little sweet cream can be beaten in before using. If used on vegetable salad the flavor is sometimes improved by the addition of a little sour cream.

Avocado Dressing

Mash very ripe avocado with fork and add a little Health Mayonnaise, or a few drops of vegetable juice, and beat until smooth and fluffy. If more seasoning is needed add a little vegetable salt and finely grated onion if the dressing is to be used for vegetable salad. If used for fruit salad, add a little honey.

We do use Apple Cider Vinegar, which is beneficial. Read the revealing chapter on Vinegar on pages 71-72 of the 1978 edition of "Fresh Vegetable and Fruit Juices" by Dr. N. W. Walker.

I never use either white sugar or white flour in any shape, manner or form as I have no desire whatever to start either an ulcer or a cancer in my system.

I never use commercial white salt because I do not want to be troubled with hardening of my arteries nor with varicose veins.

I do not use egg whites in any form because I do not want my system clogged up.

Pepper and other spicy ingredients I also omit entirely as I do not wish to have any irritation of the kidneys or bladder, nor do I want to be troubled with high blood pressure.

Swiss Cheese Dressing

Grate Swiss cheese preferably on Acme grater and add tomato juice, a few drops at a time, and thoroughly mix into cheese before adding more. Continue this until you have a dressing the consistency of thick whipped cream. This is delicious on any vegetable salad and particularly on tomatoes. It is very rich and should be used in small quantities.

Sour Cream Dressing

1 cup of sour cream, 1 teaspoonful of honey and a few drops of lemon juice whipped together until thick.

French Dressing

Olive oil (preferably cold pressed) about ½ pint, ¼ teaspoonful powdered kelp or sea lettuce, ¼ teaspoonful powdered alfalfa and a little lemon juice and honey. Thoroughly beat together until emulsified and if salt is needed add a little vegetable salt of a good quality.

* * *

A BRIEF ENCYCLOPEDIA
OF VEGETABLES, FRUITS, ETC.

It has been my experience that there is much to be gained in the long run by buying the very best vegetables and fruits in preference to those of poor quality. Even though they cost more, greater nourishment is derived from a somewhat smaller quantity of the best, than from a larger volume of poor, dried out or otherwise puny vegetables and fruits.

With present day transportation and refrigeration facilities, efficient and general as they are, there is little reason why plenty of fresh raw vegetables and fruits should not form the major part of every meal. If they do cost more in some parts of the country than in others, and if some are more scarce in certain seasons of the year, we must nevertheless bear in mind that there is a great deal more nourishing and constructive food value in a small quantity of raw vegetables than there is in a large volume of cooked foods. The former regenerate cells and tissues and furnish LIFE in the body while the latter are "fillers" without commensurate constructive value, merely sustaining life while the body disintegrates.

With rare exceptions, any vegetable or fruit which we have been accustomed to cook can be eaten raw with greater benefit. As a general rule fruits and vegetables can be mixed in salads as well as eaten separately during the same meal. Fruits act more as cleansers of the system while vegetables are builders of the cells and tissues of the body.

In the following list of the most common of our vegetables, I have indicated some of the important chemical elements they contain.

Where the *water, protein, carbohydrate,* and *fat* content are indicated, *the percentage shown is in proportion to the entire vegetable, raw.*

Where the *mineral elements, salts,* etc., are indicated, the percentage represents *their proportion in relation to the approximate total, exclusive of the water content.*

ALFALFA. This word is derived from the Arabic word meaning "best fodder." It is significant that a few generations ago carrots were considered primarily horse food while now their juice has become one of the most famous beverages in the civilized world. So alfalfa, which in the past has been the food of paramount value for cattle, will in the none too distant future supply its juice as one of the greatest aids for human ailments and deficiencies.

Only the leaves of alfalfa should be used for juice and for salads, as the fiber of the stems is very tough.

The water content of fresh alfalfa is about 80%. It is exceedingly rich in nitrogen, calcium, potassium, phosphorus and magnesium.

When fresh alfalfa is not obtainable, then the powdered can be used in salads in quantities of about one-quarter teaspoonful per portion, or in similar quantity in one pint of fresh vegetable juice.

ASPARAGUS is particularly rich in silicon, has a high phosphorus content, and a good proportion of potassium, sodium, manganese and iron. It contains more than 90% water and should be eaten in moderation as it has very strong cleansing properties, particularly for the kidneys and bladder. It should be eaten, preferably, raw as an ingredient in salads mixed with other vegetables. Cooked asparagus not only loses its nourishing value but has a tendency to irritate the kidneys.

AVOCADO (Alligator Pear) see under Fruits.

BEETS contain potassium, iron, sodium and manganese. Greater benefit is obtained when the tops as well as the roots are eaten, raw. The roots can be finely grated and the tops chopped or ground. They contain more than 87% water. The carbohydrate content is little more than 9%. The tops of beets are particularly rich in manganese which makes their iron content valuable in nourishing the liver and the red corpuscles of the blood.

Raw beets and their juices when properly extracted have been used effectively in regulating menstrual periods and premature menopause as well as constipation. It is advisable however to drink not more than a total of 8 ounces (½ pint) of straight beet juice per day until the body is able to tolerate more of it.

BROCCOLI is a food rich in potassium, phosphorus and sulphur. The stalks should be ground and used raw with the tops finely chopped. It contains approximately 90% water with a very low carbohydrate and fat content. Being a good cleanser of the body it tends to reduce excessive weight. Its very high Vitamin A content is somewhat overshadowed by its richness in sulphur and phosphorus.

BRUSSEL SPROUTS are exceedingly high in sulphur and phosphorus, rich in potassium, and the water content is approximately 85%. Due to their very high sulphur content they should be eaten sparingly. When cooked the sulphur, as well as all the other elements, are converted into inorganic substances which do more harm than good. They should be chopped finely or ground, raw, mixed with salads. They contain three times more sulphur than does cabbage.

CABBAGE. Both the red and white cabbage are valuable ingredients in a salad but only in reasonable quantities, because the sulphur and chlorine content is high. The red cabbage has a slightly tougher fiber than the white. Its chlorine, calcium and sodium content is nearly 50% more than that of the white, while on the other hand the white cabbage has about 65% more potassium, nearly ten times more iron and about three times as much silicon as the red cabbage. The water content of both is approximately 90%.

The flatulency experienced after eating cabbage is usually due to improper mastication and the presence of waste matter or debris in the stomach and intestinal tract. The cleansing effect is to stir up this debris, frequently generating an uncomfortable amount of gas in the process. When vinegar, salt or sugar is added, cabbage has a destructive effect, gravely irritating to the digestive tract.

CARROTS are undoubtedly one of our most valuable and complete foods. Finely grated they are used extensively for bulk by many who were formerly under the mistaken impression that they could not eat raw vegetables. As a matter of fact the finely grated pulp of raw carrots has been found to be one of the most soothing, efficient and beneficial means to aid the colon in nourishing itself back to a normal condition.

Raw carrots contain all the elements and all the vitamins that are required by the human body. Their value to the body however is lost when carrots are cooked, canned or otherwise processed.

Carrots that are too young are immature, the minerals and vitamins are not completely formed and they are therefore not as nourishing as when they have been allowed to grow in the ground for four and one-half to five months before being pulled.

Of the vegetable juices, raw carrot juice stands supreme, always provided that it is strictly fresh and has been properly made. It is a particularly wonderful cleanser of bile and waste matter coagulated in the liver as a result of years of wrong eating. Occasionally in some instances the skin becomes discolored, usually a yellowish hue, after drinking carrot and other juices. I have found this to be the result of the coagulated bile in the liver dissolving so fast that sluggish kidneys and bowels were not able to take care of its elimination quickly enough resulting in the lymph carrying this excess debris to the surface for elimination through the pores of the skin.

This discoloration disappears sooner or later. It is not a discoloration from the pigment of the carrot. Personally under such conditions I would much prefer a brief blow to my vanity as a result of this cleansing of the liver which would give me a much longer, healthier and active life, than to forego these life-giving juices and know that the Coroner's verdict would soon refer to the degeneration of the liver, and probably to cancer.

Bear in mind that a lifetime of wrong living, and by this I mean mainly eating the wrong kind of food, creates disintegrating processes in the body which it will take months or years to completely eradicate.

It is silly therefore to expect a miraculous regeneration of the body by merely drinking a pint of juice now and again. It is even more silly to heed the voice of ignorance when told that properly made fresh raw juices cause sickness when as a matter of fact the temporary discomfort is usually nothing more than the process of bodily "house cleaning" in a perfectly natural manner as a result of these juices. We must cooperate with Nature to undo the harm that we did to ourselves, and furnish our system regularly, daily, with the organic chemical elements in sufficient quantities with which to rebuild the cells and tissues of the body.

It takes time to do this and it is my experience that the quickest and most positive way to do it is to determine just how many pints of juices we can drink daily and strive to drink these daily without failure or exception for months or years.

Carotene is that part of the carrot which, when raw, contains the finest quality of Vitamin A that the body can assimilate. When this Vitamin is subjected to heat or other processes and concentrated, separated from the other elements furnished by Nature in the carrot, then its value is correspondingly reduced if not virtually lost. Occasionally some temporary benefit is derived from such concentrated extracts. For definite practical results nothing compares to the raw juice, when properly extracted.

Children should drink one pint of carrot juice daily. Most troubles afflicting children are recognized as due to a deficiency of Vitamin A. So is night blindness. A pint of carrot juice in the afternoon or evening is the most helpful thing I know to bring relief to eyes and reduce the fatigue resulting from driving against bright lights. It is my opinion that all drivers of busses, trucks, air pilots and others in whom the safety of lives depends during night transportation, should drink at least one pint of raw carrot juice, properly extracted, every afternoon.

Fresh carrots contain more than 87% water. About 37% of the total mineral content is potassium, with a great amount of sodium and calcium also present and a good percentage of iron, magnesium and manganese. The cleansing elements, sulphur and chlorine, are also present in ample proportions, while phosphorus, the brain food, is nearly 13%.

CAULIFLOWER is very tasty and palatable when eaten raw. It is rich in potassium while the phosphorus and sulphur contents are also high. It contains more than 90% water with a fairly high protein content. It belongs to the cabbage family and like the other members of this family has the tendency to irritate the kidneys if eaten in too large a quantity. It has good nourishing qualities however and used sparingly is a valuable addition to a salad.

CELERY. The green leaves of celery should be used whenever possible just as much as the stalks because in addition to a very high sodium content they contain also a valuable ingredient of insulin. Celery contains more than four times as much organic sodium as calcium. As the over-indulgence of concentrated starches has the tendency to leave deposits of inorganic calcium in the system, eating plenty of celery daily has been of great benefit to those afflicted with this habit. The organic sodium in the celery aids in maintaining such inorganic calcium in solution until some of it at least can be eliminated from the body before it accumulates and causes trouble. Furthermore the rich magnesium and iron content of celery furnishes valuable nourishment for the blood cells.

Celery contains nearly 95% water. It is perhaps our food richest in sodium chloride. In hot weather and in tropical climates, people who drink a lot of fresh raw celery juice do not suffer from the heat, particularly if the elimination of waste from the body is satisfactory. Common salt, which is inorganic sodium chloride, is detrimental to the system, compared to the beneficial organic sodium chloride of fresh raw celery juice.

In hot weather I make it a point to drink at least one pint a day of raw celery juice.

I have known people with nervous disorders, and afflicted with sleeplessness, to derive wonderful benefits from drinking raw celery juice. I have seen them become calm and composed, and be able to sleep, by drinking one or two glasses afternoons and evenings.

Some have discovered the sobering qualities of raw celery juice (as well as of the combination of carrot, celery, parsley and spinach juices) and have gone into its commercial production mainly to supply this as an antidote to alcoholic indulgencies.

When the root of the celery plant has been allowed to develop fully then it becomes also a valuable ingredient for salads and can be used either grated or ground. The water content of the root is 84%. The carbohydrate content is more than three times greater and potassium less than 50% that of the celery leaves and stalks. There is only a trace of sodium compared to that contained in the leaves and stalks. The iron and the silicon content also is about 50% lower.

CHICORY—see endive.

CHIVES are a pleasing addition to a salad. They belong to the onion family and contain more than 80% water. They are fairly high in protein and carbohydrate content, rich in potassium, calcium, phosphorus and sulphur. They are stimulating to the digestive system. They are valuable as a blood cleanser but exercise a strong diuretic action, consequently they should be used in moderation, particularly by those having trouble with the kidneys. People drinking beer, we find, should avoid using chives to any extent because, according to our researches, beer has a very strong disintegrating effect on the kidneys and a diuretic with the tendency to irritate the kidneys may cause undue discomfort.

CUCUMBERS are used extensively as an ingredient in nearly every meal in many hot Eastern countries such as Turkey, Egypt, etc. They are recognized as a valuable health food. Both whole cucumbers and their seeds are extensively used. They are tasty and refreshing when crisp.

Cucumbers contain more than 95% water and are very rich in potassium, iron and magnesium. They contain also a relatively high percentage of silicon and fluorine. They are therefore a very valuable food item and should be included in salads whenever possible. They may be cut into thin slices or grated.

As a food they are of great benefit to the gall bladder, the liver and the kidneys. Their high silicon and fluorine content makes them a valuable food also for the hair, teeth and nails.

Cucumbers should be peeled. Passing the tongs of a fork along the length of the cucumber all the way around it, breaking the skin, makes it seemingly easier to masticate and more readily digested.

DANDELION. Dandelion greens contain more than 85% water. They are very rich in potassium, calcium, sodium and particularly magnesium. The acid elements are low, giving the composition of this plant a close relation to the alkaline-acid percentage in the human body. It is very rich in most of the vitamins, particularly in A, B, C and D. The dandelion flower is very rich in Vitamin D.

Dandelion has a very stimulating effect on the glands. Its principle value is in nourishing the bone structure of the body, particularly giving strength and firmness to the teeth. It is valuable also in stimulating lymph activity, thus aiding elimination through the pores of the skin.

The whole plant, leaves, flowers and roots can be used, both in salads and in making juice. Because of its bitter taste it is advisable to use the juice mixed with carrot juice thereby also adding the valuable constructive elements of the carrot as a base.

ENDIVE and other varieties of the chicory plant are all valuable ingredients for salads. They are somewhat bitter and this tends to stimulate the secretion of saliva. By promoting also the secretion of bile it aids in cleansing the liver. It stimulates the activity of the spleen. It contains about 90% water but the fibers are somewhat tough and should therefore be chewed thoroughly.

Rich in potassium, sodium, calcium and phosphorus, the juice of endive, particularly when added to the juices of carrots, celery and parsley, is very nourishing to the optic system. I have known of many instances in which people with eye trouble have been able to discard their glasses after a few months when drinking these juices regularly. As a matter of fact we have on record the case of a woman whose total blindness of more than two years' duration was relieved to such an extent that in the course of a few months she was able to read a newspaper with a magnifying glass, as a result of drinking this combination and other raw juices daily, in addition to changing her diet.

FENNEL is a very valuable vegetable used in large quantities by the Latin races. As its nourishing value is becoming better known it is gradually becoming a more popular addition to other raw vegetables, either in salads or as a side dish. Fennel contains nearly 90% water in the bulbous part of the plant, which is the edible part.

This vegetable can be either quartered, sliced, chopped or ground. It is a very alkalinizing food, aiding in loosening up mucous or phlegm conditions, besides helping to stimulate the digestive processes. It is a good diuretic. It has a high sodium content and is rich in potassium and iron.

GARLIC has a beneficial effect on the lymph, aiding in the elimination of noxious waste matter in the body, having the tendency to increase body-odor until such waste has been sufficiently eliminated. It is a valuable cleanser of the mucous membranes, particularly the lungs, the sinuses, the nose and the throat. For this reason it is a valuable food in pulmonary conditions, asthma, etc.

Although occasionally somewhat irritating to the kidneys, garlic is nevertheless valuable for its diuretic action. It is also a useful cleanser of the blood therefore helpful in conditions of high blood pressure. It tends to stimulate peristaltic action and the secretion of digestive juices.

While the odor of garlic is not usually appreciated as a second hand perfume, this condition can be compensated by the use of raw parsley, mint or other fresh green herbs of a like nature, combined with it, or used immediately afterwards.

Garlic contains approximately 65% water and satisfactory results are obtained by using it raw, chopped finely, in small quantities as an ingredient in any vegetable salad.

HORSERADISH is one of our most valuable concentrated, natural foods, in that it contains one of the most efficient solvents of mucus, or phlegm, in the system, particularly that in the sinuses and nasal cavities, due to a peculiar quality of highly penetrating ether of the mustard oil nature. This applies to the horseradish root, when ground, or preferably triturated, and taken in quantities of not more than one-half teaspoonful at a time, because while it stimulates the appetite and aids in the secretion of digestive juices, it has a tendency to irritate the kidneys and the bladder if taken in larger quantities.

It contains more than 75% water and of its mineral contents, 30% is potassium while 29% is sulphur. The acid elements in horseradish are about 10% higher than the alkaline elements.

KALE belongs to the cabbage family and contains more than 90% water. It is particularly rich in sulphur, phosphorus, and chlorine, while potassium represents more than 30% of the total mineral elements. It is valuable as a cleanser but has a tendency to generate gas when the condition of the system is over-acid. It is rich in vitamins and the plant should be eaten when young because the fibers become tough when the plant is old.

LEEKS belong to the onion family and contain more than 90% water. They are rich in potassium and calcium, having also a fair volume of phosphorus, chlorine and sulphur. They are rich in vitamins B and C.

They are good cleansers of the system, aiding in the stimulation of the pancreas and in the secretion of digestive juices. They are cleansers of the blood stream and stimulating to the muscles in their action when they are overloaded with uric acid due to the frequent or large consumption of meat.

They should be used not merely as a condiment in salads but in sufficient quantity to make them an important ingredient thereof.

LETTUCE. The various varieties of lettuce constitute one of our most valuable foods because of their large organic water content, ranging from 92 to 95 per cent, and on account of the abundance of potassium, sodium, calcium and, particularly, magnesium and iron they contain. They are also rich in those essential elements, silicon and fluorine.

When eaten raw without the addition of condiments or seasoning, lettuce of every kind is one of the most nourishing foods for the cells and tissues of the nervous and muscular structures of the body. Nearly all the necessary vitamins are found in lettuce and this vegetable rates third highest in value, carrot being first, alfalfa second. The outer leaves of lettuce are the most valuable, as these contain most of the vital nourishing elements. Whenever possible, lettuce should be an important ingredient in every salad because of its potent effect in stimulating metabolism.

The raw juice of lettuce turns almost black when separated from the pulp. With the addition of carrot juice it is a valuable aid in digestion where stomach ulcers would otherwise interfere with the digestive processes. Lettuce can be used in salads either in chunks or chopped in whatever size is desired.

SEA LETTUCE is a marine plant, like kelp, furnishing one of our richest supplies of organic iodine. It is usually obtained in finely ground or powdered form and due to its high potency should not be used in greater quantities than one-fourth teaspoonful daily, preferably mixed with a pint of raw vegetable juice.

A combination of carrot, celery, parsley and spinach, the richest natural potassium combination, and the addition of one-fourth teaspoonful of powdered Sea Lettuce, thoroughly mixed, has furnished aid and comfort to troublesome conditions of the thyroid gland, as in goiter, by enabling the body to assimilate this nourishment through the blood stream readily and very quickly.

MUSTARD GREENS have a high sulphur, phosphorus and chlorine content and a fairly large percentage of other mineral elements, particularly potassium. The water content is more than 85% and this vegetable is therefore a good cleansing food, particularly if the leaves are young.

They have somewhat of a laxative effect on some people. Eaten raw in moderate amounts they form a valuable ingredient for a salad.

NETTLES are not a very popular vegetable because of the stiff prickly hairs which cover the leaves. They are, however, a valuable nourishing food and they are better prepared by passing them through a food chopper using a coarse blade. They help to bring out the flavor and enhance the value of any salad in which they are included.

They are rich in vitamins and their potassium, calcium and sodium content is high.

The water content when the plant is young is nearly 90%.

OKRA when eaten raw is particularly valuable as a food for those who are troubled with inflammation of the intestines. By itself, okra is a somewhat slimy food to eat raw, but one or two ground up with spinach or mustard greens, or lettuce leaves, added to a salad forms a valuable ingredient for the secretion of digestive juices and has a soothing effect on irritations of the colon, bladder and kidneys.

The water content of okra is more than 90%. The calcium content is more than one-third that of all its combined mineral elements, while the sodium content is approximately 20%.

ONIONS are rich in ether oils which have very penetrating qualities, beneficial to the mucous membrane. Some varieties are stronger than others in this respect, the stronger being used mainly for condiments while some of the larger variety whose flavor is not quite so penetrating are more frequently used as a food ingredient in salads.

They are rich in carbohydrates. About 25% of the mineral elements is potassium, while calcium, silicon, phosphorus and iron are also abundant. The water content is in excess of 85%.

PARSLEY is one of the most potent foods of the common vegetable kingdom. As a juice, if properly and completely extracted, it is not wise to drink more than ¼ pint (4 ounces) daily without the addition of other vegetable juices because otherwise it is likely to create a serious disturbance of the nervous system. With the addition of the raw juice of carrots and celery it is very valuable as nourishment for the optic system, also for the kidneys and bladder and as an aid in allaying inflammation of the urethra and genital organs. It stimulates the secretion of digestive juices and helps considerably in disturbances of the liver and of the spleen.

The water content of parsley is in excess of 85% but the fibers are so tough that it requires a very thorough trituration and a sufficient amount of hydraulic pressure to extract all of the vitamins and mineral elements with the juice.

Parsley is rich in potassium, calcium, magnesium and chlorine. In salads it should be ground up very fine and can be used to the extent of one to two tablespoons per serving, not merely to decorate it.

When eating meat, raw parsley should be eaten at the same time, because of its diuretic action, in order to stimulate the elimination of the excessive uric acid resulting from the digestion of meat.

PARSNIPS contain more than 80% water and are fairly rich in carbohydrates. Of the mineral elements they contain more than 40% potassium, nearly 10% silicon and are also rich in phosphorus, sulphur and chlorine. They have a fairly active effect on the urinary system and are helpful in conditions of bladder, and kidney stones. The tops are rich in mineral elements but care should be taken to avoid the wild variety as these contain certain poisons which are very detrimental to the human system.

The whole plant of the cultivated variety can be used to advantage ground, grated or chopped in salads.

PEAS when fresh are an excellent vegetable but when dried come under the classification of legumes. Fresh peas are of much greater value as an item of food when eaten raw in salads than when cooked. They are rich in potassium and magnesium. The pods of young fresh peas can be used to advantage in salads by removing the stem and stringy parts.

As a juice the fresh peas, including the pods, contain an ingredient which aids the pancreas in its functions. When fresh, peas contain nearly 75% water and a little more than 15% carbohydrate, while the dried peas contain only about 15% water, but the carbohydrate content is nearly 55% and the protein about 23%.

PEPPERS. Green peppers as well as the sweet red and yellow peppers are particularly valuable because of their high silicon and fluorine content which furnish very necessary nourishment for the skin, nails and hair. They contain more than 90% water.

They can be used sliced, chopped or grated in salads and, when properly extracted, their juice added to carrot juice makes a very valuable nourishing drink.

Hot peppers are irritants and overstimulating to the digestive tract, particularly to the intestines, kidneys and bladder.

POTATOES when raw contain more than 75% water, about 20% carbohydrate and a small percentage of very valuable protein. They are very rich in potassium which represents 60% of their total mineral elements. They are rich in Vitamins A, B and C. As a matter of fact few vegetables contain as much Vitamin C as raw potatoes. They should be eaten raw with the skin, and in salads they can be grated or sliced.

When the potato is cooked the value of the mineral elements and most of the vitamins is lost. The water content is reduced to approximately 10% while the carbohydrate content is increased to more than 65%. The raw potato contains a sugary carbohydrate which is readily digested, whereas upon cooking this is converted into a starchy carbohydrate which leaves an acid end product in the process of digestion. This is particularly the case when they are eaten during the same meal with concentrated proteins.

Potatoes that are fried in fat are not only indigestible but also have a tendency to create a disturbance of the liver and gall bladder.

Sweet potatoes contain a little less water and about 20% more carbohydrates than the Irish variety. Their potassium content however is lower while the sodium, calcium, silicon and chlorine content is considerably higher. This applies to sweet potatoes when raw. When cooked they are affected in a similar manner as the Irish potato.

PUMPKINS contain about 90% water with a comparatively low percentage of carbohydrates. While rich in sodium, potassium, magnesium and iron, they are rich also in chlorine and phosphorus. They have laxative qualities and their diuretic properties do not irritate the kidneys.

Raw pumpkin is delicious when very finely grated and served in combination with finely grated carrots, beets, etc., as a base for salads. To cook pumpkins destroys their valuable water content, reducing it to about 15% and increases the carbohydrate content to more than 50%, converting it from a sugar to a starchy carbohydrate.

RADISHES. These may be considered under the general classification of large and small radishes. The former contain a little more than 85% water, but 50% less mineral elements than the small, while the latter contain more than 93% water and are rich in potassium, sodium and calcium with a large percentage of chlorine. They are rich also in phosphorus and sulphur while the large variety is particularly rich in silicon.

Radishes contain a volatile ether which has a particular affinity for mucus or phlegm as a solvent thereof. They have also enzymes valuable in aiding the secretion of digestive juices. Because of their diuretic action they are valuable in cleansing the kidneys and the bladder.

The juice of radishes blended with carrot juice is a wonderful aid in cleansing and healing the mucous membrane of the digestive system as well as of the respiratory organs.

The small radishes are used either whole or sliced to garnish salads, while the large radishes can be grated or shredded as an ingredient.

RUTABAGAS are particularly valuable as an ingredient in salads because of the pre-eminence of Vitamins B and C, as well as a small quantity of Vitamin A. They are particularly rich in potassium and contain more than 88% water.

In general they resemble turnips in physical characteristics and physiological effects.

SAUERKRAUT is a preparation of pickled cabbage. The cabbage is cut into fine shreds, placed in layers with salt in abundant quantities, pepper and other spices are sometimes added, and it is then allowed to ferment. It furnishes a food which may be appetizing to the palate but is destructive to the digestive system because of the presence of the unnatural ferments and large quantities of inorganic salt. Such salt tends to deplete the vitality of blood vessels and to stimulate other degenerative processes in the system.

SPINACH is one of the most valuable of our leafy vegetables. It contains more than 88% water and is particularly rich in the finest quality of organic iron obtainable. It is also rich in sodium, potassium and calcium, while the magnesium content is very high.

The juice of this vegetable, when raw and fresh, is one of the most nourishing foods for the entire digestive and particularly the eliminative organs. While cathartics and laxatives operate as a result of irritation of the lower intestines, spinach juice follows the natural course of nourishing the cells and tissues as well as nerves and muscles so that eventually normal elimination may be established. The addition of fresh raw carrot juice to spinach juice is a particularly good aid to re-establish the normal tone of the intestines.

Spinach contains a valuable quality of oxalic acid. When the spinach is raw this oxalic acid in its natural form is organic and in combination with the other natural elements present in the spinach, stimulates the peristaltic action of the intestines. When spinach is cooked however the organic principle of all of the elements is destroyed and this applies equally to the oxalic acid, which is then converted into an inorganic acid and as such has the tendency to form oxalic acid crystals in the kidneys.

In salads, raw spinach should be added as an important ingredient. After washing thoroughly, the leaves can either be chopped fine or ground through a machine of the meat grinder type, using the coarsest possible knife. After one has become accustomed to eating it raw in this manner, its flavor and value is usually more fully appreciated than that of the cooked spinach.

SQUASH is a member of the melon family. The pumpkin is likewise a member of this family and its general description applies very closely to all the varieties of squash.

Squash can be eaten raw to better advantage than when cooked and for salads it can be prepared in the same manner as described for pumpkins.

TOMATOES are a fruit. See them described in the list of fruits.

TURNIPS are of two principal varieties most commonly used as a table vegetable, the white and the yellow. The yellow type has a much stronger flavor than the white.

Turnips contain nearly 90% water and of the mineral content nearly 50% is potassium. The leaves contain an exceedingly high percentage of calcium and are very rich in iron, magnesium and potassium.

The tops together with the roots are particularly valuable when converted into juice. In this manner they are an excellent food for every part of the bone structure of the body. By combining the juice of turnip leaves with carrot and dandelion juice, we have a means of effectively nourishing the bone structure of the body, particularly the teeth, in adults no less than in children.

In a salad, turnip leaves are somewhat difficult to handle unless passed through a machine of the meat chopping type as described in the preparation of spinach. Turnip roots can be grated, shredded or ground as a valuable ingredient in salads.

WATERCRESS is one of our foods richest in sulphur. It is also rich in potassium, calcium, sodium and magnesium, as well as phosphorus and chlorine. It is therefore a powerful cleanser. The water content is in excess of 92%.

In salads it can be used either in its natural state or finely chopped, either as a garnish or an ingredient.

Raw watercress juice freshly made is usually too strong to be taken alone. When combined with carrot, spinach and turnip leaves juice, a combination is obtained which has proved to be a valuable cleanser of the blood stream. It has been used effectively as an aid to dissolve the coagulated fibrin in the blood vessels which causes hemorrhoids and certain other tumorous formations.

FRUITS (FRESH)

Fruits are the cleansers of the body. They contain 75% to more than 90% water and while the protein content is low the carbohydrate content is correspondingly higher.

Raw fruits contain no starch. It is only when they are cooked that the sugar carbohydrates in some of them is converted into a starchy carbohydrate. In the process of digestion these starchy carbohydrates must be re-converted into primary sugars before they can be used in the body, usually overtaxing those organs, such as the pancreas, whose function it is to aid in this conversion.

It is the high carbon content of fruits that causes them to be the cleansers of the body. Figuratively speaking, this carbon serves to incinerate waste matter in the body but this only takes place when the fruits are fresh and raw, and also provided that no concentrated sugar or starch is eaten during the same meal when fruits are eaten. When concentrated starches and sugars are included in a meal in which fresh, raw fruits (with the exception of bananas, dates, figs and raisins) are present then the fruits no longer have an alkaline reaction in the body but tend to create an acid condition, at the same time causing the carbohydrates to ferment.

APPLES, when eaten on an empty stomach, tend to stimulate the activities of the lower intestines. They are rich in magnesium, iron and silicon, while their potassium content is very high. They contain approximately 85% water and are a valuable aid to digestion, both in their natural state and in the form of fresh juice.

There are a great many varieties of apples, the Delicious being the mildest and usually the easiest to digest. Apples have a cleansing effect which is particularly noticeable when impactions are present in the intestines and in this condition during the cleansing process some varieties are likely to give some discomfort. When this is the case then it is sometimes found that some other varieties may be eaten with less or no discomfort.

The juice of fresh apples, when raw, is of great help in the case of fevers and inflammation. Apple cider has a beneficial effect on the system.

Fresh raw apple juice is frequently classed as "sweet" cider. We have covered the subject of Vinegar quite fully on page 71 of the 1978 Revised Enlarged Edition of the book *FRESH VEGETABLE AND FRUIT JUICES, What's Missing in Your Body?* by Dr. N. W.

Walker. It is strongly recommended that you read and study that chapter before using Vinegar. This is very important.

Apples may be eaten in their natural state, whole, with any vegetables and concentrated proteins, as well as with other fruits.

As a top dressing for salads they can be grated or shredded. In like manner they make a delicious base for any fruit meal.

No sugar of any kind should ever be added to apples. If sweetening is needed, then honey should be used.

APRICOTS are one of our most delicate fruits. Due to the perishable quality of their texture, they are difficult to ship. Tree ripened apricots are one of the finest sources of organic iron for the building up of the red corpuscles of the blood. Silicon is another very valuable element found in apricots.

The water content of apricots is approximately 85%, when ripe.

When cooked the vital quality of this fruit is destroyed. When fresh and ripe they are a delectable addition to a salad, whether fruit or vegetable. As a dessert they may be eaten alone or with any other fruits.

AVOCADO, also known as Alligator Pear, contains more than 70% water. It is one of our most valuable sources of supply of organic fat, which forms 20% of its composition. It is fairly rich in mineral matter and should not be eaten until it is ripe, at which time it is mellow and its texture has the semi-soft consistency of butter. As a matter of fact it can be used raw in the place of butter.

Avocado is an exceptionally nutritious food and should be used daily whenever obtainable. On salads it can be halved, sliced diagonally, or in rings and added either as an integral part of the salad or as a garnish. It can also be whipped to a creamy consistency and flavored with lemon juice, onion juice, garlic, etc., and used as a salad dressing on either fruit or vegetable salads.

The fruit is ripe when the flesh will yield gently to a slight pressure of the fingers.

BANANAS should be eaten only when absolutely

ripe, in which state no green whatever is showing on any part, particularly at the ends. When ripe, bananas contain more than 75% water, while the carbohydrate sugar content is 22% but this is not completely formed until they are ripe. They are rich in potassium; also in sodium and magnesium.

Either cold or excessive heat will prevent their maturing satisfactorily.

When bananas are ripe they are particularly sensitive to low temperatures. Placing them in a cold refrigerator will turn them black and may spoil their flavor. To prevent deterioration they should be kept at a temperature of a little more than 50° F.

In selecting bananas, those which are full and plump will be found generally to have more flavor and delicacy, although some varieties of an inferior quality taste flat even though they may be plump.

Bananas are a carbohydrate fruit, but as the large sugar carbohydrate content is of a natural quality, and the percentage of water is high, they are readily digested, when ripe, and are compatible when mixed with other fruits.

BERRIES, including blackberries, gooseberries, huckleberries, raspberries and strawberries as well as all other varieties of edible berries, are valuable nutritional foods with great cleansing properties. They all contain a high percentage of water ranging approximately from 80% to nearly 90%.

All berries are rich in potassium and other mineral elements and when ripe, contain valuable natural sugars which are an aid in cleansing the system.

When sweetening is required, honey should be used on berries. They should never be sweetened with sugar of any kind, because they will then cause fermentation in the system, resulting in an acid reaction. This is also the case when berries are added to cereals, cakes, pies and other starchy foods. A similar acid reaction then takes place in the body.

The juice of berries is particularly beneficial to the system when taken raw. That value however is considerably lost when the juices have been canned or in any way preserved, in which state their life principle has been destroyed, and the elements have become inorganic.

Cranberries, unlike other berries, are considerably more acid and are therefore covered in a subsequent paragraph under CRANBERRIES, which see.

CHERRIES are nearly 80% water and are rich in natural fruit sugars as well as mineral elements.

The dark cherries are of more value to the system than the light colored ones, containing, as they do, a greater quantity of magnesium and iron, and much silicon. They are valuable as blood cleansers, they stimulate the secretion of digestive juices and of the urine. They are effective cleansers of the liver and kidneys.

When in season a whole meal can be made of nothing but good ripe cherries, to the extent of one or two pounds per meal.

CRANBERRIES contain nearly 90% water. Their sulphur content is exceedingly high. They also contain large quantities of certain acids, particularly oxalic and tannic acids. Their reaction on the body is consequently distinctly acid and this is considerably aggravated when they are cooked, particularly with the addition of sugar.

Under certain conditions, raw cranberries are beneficial, as for example, in kidney and liver disturbances, and sometimes in excessive looseness of the bowels.

Due to their excessive acidity however they are a fruit best used with utmost discretion if not eliminated entirely from the diet.

CURRANTS. The most common varieties are red, white and black currants. They contain approximately 80% water and are rich in potassium. Their carbohydrate content is about 11% in the red, 13% in the white and nearly 19% in the black. The red have a much higher proportion of the acid elements. They are however all beneficial in stimulating the secretion of various glands. The fresh raw juice of currants is valuable especially to the kidneys and in inflammatory conditions of the body. They are also an aid in alleviating mucous conditions of the intestinal tract.

When currants are cooked, and particularly when sugar is added, their beneficial value is lost. When used as a jelly or a jam in connection with concentrated carbohydrates, or starches, they are very acid forming.

DATES are one of the fruits richest in natural carbohydrates. The water content of dates is comparatively low, while the carbohydrate content, in the form of natural sugars, is about 70%. They are rich in potassium and chlorine and their general alkaline content is high.

Dates are one of the most valuable substitutes for candy. Adults, no less than children, should be encouraged to eat these in the place of candies which are excessively acid-forming.

Care should be taken to avoid eating dates which have been treated with sulphuric acid to preserve them. Fortunately this method is gradually falling into disuse.

Dates are very useful to use in the place of bread and other starches. They are beneficial, and not acid-forming.

Their carbohydrate is composed of natural sugars and they are compatible therefore with other fruits.

Date Sugar is a product of the natural crystallization of the carbohydrates in dates. It is a very good substitute for cane or other sugars and a good quality can be readily obtained at the best health food stores. It can be used freely as an adjunct to vegetable and fruit salads. It is also delicious on fruit with cream for breakfast.

FIGS. Fresh figs, both of the white and the dark variety, are exceedingly beneficial, being in fact one of the best natural laxatives. They contain nearly 80% water and have a very high potassium, calcium and magnesium content.

When in season fresh figs should be eaten in abundance, particularly by children.

GRAPES contain on an average about 80% water. Their sugar carbohydrate is high but they do not come under the carbohydrate fruit classification. They are very rich in potassium and iron and have a predominance of alkaline elements.

Fresh ripe grapes in season are among our most wholesome fruits, being one of the greatest aids in the elimination of uric acid from the system. They are also valuable because they stimulate the secretion of digestive juices.

The extensive use of grapes as an eliminative diet has become a popular and successful method towards re-establishing the alkaline-acid chemical balance of the body. Grapes of every variety have proved valuable for this purpose.

A meal composed entirely of grapes, say about one or two pounds, according to the taste or capacity of the individual, is generally very satisfying and sustaining. It is frequently found that eating about one-half pound of ripe grapes every two hours throughout the day for three or four days, omitting all other food, has a beneficial, cleansing effect on the whole system.

GRAPEFRUIT has proved to be one of the most valuable fruits as an aid in the removal or dissolving of inorganic calcium which may have formed deposits in the cartilage of the joints, as in Arthritis, as a result of an excessive consumption of devitalized white flour products. Fresh grapefruit contains organic salicylic acid which aids in dissolving such inorganic calcium in the body.

It is also rich in other fruit acids and sugars. It contains nearly 87% water and is rich in potassium and other alkaline elements.

Sugar should never be added to grapefruit because the acids cause a fermentation of the sugar in the system and the fruit will then tend to have an acid, instead of an alkaline reaction in the body.

When grapefruit or its juice has been canned or in any way preserved, the value of the organic elements is lost and the acids are converted into inorganic acids of little value to the body.

LEMONS are very rich in organic citric acid, and, while acid to the taste, they have a powerful alkaline reaction on the body, provided that no sugar is added. They contain nearly 90% water.

Lemon juice is a wonderful natural antiseptic for cuts, etc. It may sting a little at first, but not really painfully.

The juice of lemons without the addition of sugar is one of the most valuable aids we have. For example, I have known many to take the juice of two lemons in 4 ounces of hot water every hour or two for one or two days, omitting all other food during that time and so break down and eliminate an aggravated cold. In like manner lemon juice has been used successfully as an aid in a great many other conditions of bodily discomfort or chemical unbalance.

The use of bicarbonate of soda in lemonade generates gas.

LIMES are the product of a cross between lemons and oranges and while sweeter than the former they partake of the properties and qualities of both. As a matter of fact when still green they are sometimes used in the place of lemons while the ripe ones are occasionally used instead of oranges. It is best to use them only when ripe.

MELONS, including all the varieties, are extremely beneficial, particularly when forming the entire meal. When eating melons it is best not to eat any other food during the same meal, but to eat all the melon one desires.

The water content of melons ranges from 90 to 93% according to the variety. They have a small proportion of cellulose fiber which is readily digested if no other food is present to interfere with their digestion. They are rich in potassium and the percentage of alkaline elements is in proportion of three to one of the acid elements.

They are particularly desirable for kidney disorders on account of their valuable diuretic action. In some cases the addition of a little lemon juice is beneficial but neither sugar nor salt should be added to them.

These paragraphs apply in a general way to cantaloupes, casabas, honey dew, muskmelon, persians, watermelons, etc.

NECTARINES, when ripe, contain nearly 83% water. Their composition is very similar to that of the peach, being rich in potassium with a fair percentage of calcium and sodium. They have however a higher carbohydrate content than peaches. They are good cleansers and have a delectable flavor. When ripe the stone is freely removable.

OLIVES are particularly rich in fat. They contain more than 50% fat as against nearly 40% water. They are exceptionally rich in potassium which represents more than 80% of all the combined water-free minerals and salts.

Ripe olives are a healthy food furnishing the body with a valuable lubricant.

ORANGES contain nearly 87% water and are rich in potassium, calcium and magnesium. They also contain silicon. The organic citric acids and other fruit acid salts combine to make this one of our most valuable fruits.

They are very rich in Vitamins A, B and C.

There are few fruits whose alkaline effect on an over-acid condition of the body, is so rapid. It is frequently one of the most valuable fruits to use during a fruit fast, when a diet of oranges and orange juice alone, in abundant quantities daily, to the exclusion of all other foods, for three to six days, has proved extremely beneficial.

From babyhood to senility, no fruit has been known to have more generally far reaching effects than oranges and their juice. So long as they are available they should be used daily, either during or between meals.

Oranges should be used within fifteen minutes from the time they are opened because they oxidize so rapidly.

Under no circumstances should sugar in any shape or form be added as a sweetening. If any sweetening is desired honey should be used.

PAPAYAS are of particular value because of their protein digestive elements. They are therefore valuable to stimulate the appetite and the secretion of the digestive juices. They are a tropical fruit, rich in sodium and magnesium as well as phosphorus and sulphur, and their water content is in excess of 87%.

PEACHES contain more than 88% water and are rich in potassium, calcium and sodium. They are easily digested, have a strong alkaline reaction on the body, and stimulate the secretion of the digestive juices.

They have both laxative and diuretic qualities and are an aid in cleansing the system in kidney and bladder trouble.

When peaches are cooked or canned their vital elements are lost. When sugar is added the reaction in the body is acid. Sugar should not be used with peaches. If sweetening is needed, the use of honey is recommended.

PEARS contain nearly 85% water and are very rich in alkaline elements. They have a strong diuretic action and are valuable as general cleansers of the system.

When cooked, canned or processed their greatest value is lost, the organic elements being thereby converted into inorganic matter.

PERSIMMONS contain more than 66% water with

a rich carbohydrate content. They should not be eaten until fully ripened because only then have the sugars been completely formed. They are rich in potassium and magnesium with a percentage of phosphorus which is more pronounced before the fruit is ripe. They are noted for their laxative qualities.

PINEAPPLES contain nearly 90% water and are rich in potassium, calcium and sodium. Due to the fairly large amount of sulphur and chlorine which is also present, they are valuable cleansers.

Pineapples contain a fair amount of acids, notably citric, malic and tartaric, which in their organic form are an aid to digestion and exert a diuretic action.

Although the organic elements lose their vital qualities in the process of preserving or canning, nevertheless certain temporary benefits are derived from the use of these, provided that no sugar whatever has been added to them.

As a top dressing for salads, sliced or crushed pineapple, preferably raw, is a palatable addition, and beneficial, provided that it has not been sweetened with sugar.

PLUMS contain more than 78% water and are rich in potassium, calcium, magnesium and phosphorus. They contain several fruit acids some of which have a tendency to irritate the kidneys. They have, however, a strong laxative action. Plums are best eaten raw and ripe in which state they are sweet and juicy and the stone is readily removed.

This applies to all varieties of plums, including greengages, damsons, beech plums, etc.

POMEGRANATE contains nearly 77% water and is exceptionally rich in sodium which represents nearly 50% of all the combined mineral elements and salts. It contains some Vitamin A and is rich in Vitamins B and C.

The skin and partitions of the pomegranate have a very high tannic acid content and other bitter ingredients and have a constipating effect. The edible parts however have a cleansing and cooling effect on the system generally and are somewhat laxative.

The juice of pomegranates, either straight or with the addition of fresh raw carrot juice or with apple juice, makes a very healthful and pleasing beverage.

QUINCES are only fit to eat when tree-ripened in

warm climates, at which time the natural fruit sugars have matured. When used green, in an unripened state, and with the addition of sugar, they are very acid-forming in the system.

RHUBARB is one of the most detrimental foods due to the exceedingly high oxalic acid content. The addition of sugar when cooking it aggravates its acid-forming qualities. It seems to me to be an utterly unnecessary addition to a diet, because of its pernicious effect. (Read the chapter on Oxalic Acid in the book *FRESH VEGETABLE AND FRUIT JUICES, What's Missing in Your Body?*)

TOMATOES are a fruit of the acid variety, having a strong alkaline reaction on the system provided that no concentrated sugary or starchy carbohydrate is present while eating them or during the period of their digestion. The addition of sugar, bread or crackers, etc., causes fermentation and much acidity in the digestive system.

Tomatoes contain 94% water and are exceedingly rich in potassium, magnesium, sodium and calcium. They are also high in chlorine and phosphorus with a small percentage of silicon.

In their natural state, fresh, ripe and raw, they are extremely beneficial, having a very rapid alkaline reaction on the system. They can be eaten whole, sliced or quartered in salads and their fresh raw juice is particularly cleansing and vitalizing.

The addition of spices and of preservatives such as Benzoate of Soda, etc., completely destroys the beneficial effects of this fruit, causing instead irritations of the intestines, kidneys, etc.

One of the frequent causes of ulcerations in the intestinal tract among the Latin races has been attributed to the excessive use of tomatoes in combination with concentrated starch products, such as breads, macaroni and spaghetti of all kinds, rice, etc., and it is interesting to know that these ulcerated conditions have been relieved when these incompatible combinations were eliminated from the diet.

Tomatoes which have been cooked, canned or processed in any manner, have lost their principal organic value.

DRIED FRUITS

When fresh fruits are not available it is an advantage to be able to obtain sun-dried fruits which have not been sulphured or processed in any way. The purpose of sulphuring dried fruits is to improve their keeping qualities, and sometimes to enhance their appearance. In this process the fruit is thoroughly impregnated with inorganic sulphur which cannot be washed completely out of the fruit. It is therefore preferable to choose those dried fruits which have not been processed in this manner.

Generally speaking, great benefits may be derived from dried fruits, particularly when the fresh fruits are not available. In the process of drying or dessicating, the water content is reduced to approximately one-fifth of that of the fresh fruit. The natural sugar carbohydrates, in the form of fruit sugars, are correspondingly increased to about five times the percentage contained in the fresh fruit.

The most satisfactory way to use dried fruits is to wash them thoroughly and place them in a dish barely covering them with distilled water, leaving them to soak long enough to permit them to become soft but not soggy, before using. If all the water has not become absorbed in the fruit, it is an indication that too much water was used.

The fruits should then be kept chilled until used.

NUTS

Nuts are among our most valuable supplies of concentrated proteins and fats. By eating one pound, to one and a half pounds of unsalted raw nuts a week, I have found that meat is not necessary as a food, even when doing heavy manual labor, particularly when starches and sugars also are omitted, using in their place an abundance of raw fruits and vegetables, and of course, a sufficient quantity of raw vegetable juices.

ALMONDS, when fresh, raw and unsalted, are the most alkaline of all nuts, being particularly valuable as nourishment for the bone structure of the body, and especially for strengthening the enamel of the teeth.

Next in the order of their greater value, are pecans, pignolias (pine nuts), black walnuts, butternuts, beechnuts, English walnuts, filberts, the rest following as of average value.

It is a mistake to eat nuts at the end of a meal, particularly at the end of a heavy meal, because they are a highly concentrated NATURAL food with a large percentage of fat and protein in their composition, and therefore require a fairly free digestive system for the body to obtain the utmost benefit from them. Eaten in small quantities between meals, particularly when drinking fresh raw carrot juice, they are particularly beneficial.

CASHEW nuts are not as readily digested as the others. They belong more closely to the Legumes.

PEANUTS are not nuts. They are one of the Legumes most destructive to the human system on account of their extremely acid action not only on the digestive system but on the whole body. There are few things people eat that are so destructive as peanuts. They rank second only to popcorn in their pernicious effect. Read the following chapter on Legumes.

NUTS which have been cooked, roasted, or otherwise subjected to excessive heat, are harmful on account of the change which takes place in the fat under these conditions. The reaction on the liver and gall bladder is then detrimental and may sooner or later interfere with the complete and proper function of these organs.

NUT BUTTERS are sometimes more readily digested than the nuts themselves provided that neither the nuts nor the butters have been subjected to heat.

CHESTNUTS usually contain as high as 50 to 75% carbohydrates.

LEGUMES

Beans of every kind, except string beans, as well as lentils, peas and corn, *when dried*, are exceedingly acid-forming because of the very low organic water content and the high percentage of concentrated protein and carbohydrates present. Human beings, while able to tolerate this combination for a while, do not have the same "mechanics" that we find in the digestion of cattle, for which legumes are a natural food. While cattle thrive on this food, the human body is sooner or later beset with the acidity of excessive fermentation and putrefaction caused by this incompatible combination. This applies no less to the flour products of legumes. Soy bean is no exception to this fundamental, natural law.

When legumes are raw and strictly fresh, then their water content ranges between 65% and 85%, and the protein and carbohydrate content is closer to the proportions found in fresh vegetables and fruits. They may be eaten raw, in salads, making an interesting and palatable addition thereto.

FOOD CONTROL GUIDE

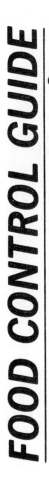

PROTEINS

Nuts
Poultry
Goats Milk
Eggs, Fish
Cheese

No

Yes

Yes

VEGETABLES

Artichokes, Asparagus, String Beans, Beets
Fresh Lima Beans, Brussels Sprouts, Okra
Lettuce, Olives, Onions, Salsify, Squash
Cabbage, Carrots, Cauliflower, Cucumber
Parsnips, Fresh Green Peas, Radishes
Celery, Dandelion Greens, Egg Plant
Swiss Chard, Turnips, Watercress
Rutabagas, Sauerkraut, Spinach

Yes

No

FRUITS

Prunes
Apricots
Cherries
Grapefruit
Nectarines
Blackberries
Lemons, Pears
Currants, Grapes
Oranges, Peaches
Rhubarb, Pineapple
Apples, Watermelon
Tomatoes, Strawberries
Raspberries, Tangerines

120

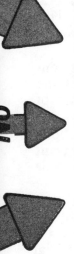

CARBOHYDRATES
(SUGAR AND STARCH)

> All cold cereals and breakfast foods, popcorn, macaroni, bread, cake, cookies, (flour products), candy, all sugars and syrups.

Note:
Use honey for
all sweetening

With meals containing starches and sugars use only these fruits: bananas, dates, figs and raisins.

Use this for your daily guide:

Do not eat any concentrated carbohydrate foods during a meal in which acid or semi-acid fruits or concentrated proteins are included.

No means: *Do not combine these foods during the same meal.*
Yes means: *These foods may be eaten together.*

FRESH VEGETABLE AND FRUIT JUICES,
What's Missing In Your Body?
By N. W. Walker, D. Sc.

New, Revised and Enlarged Edition

If we are well, we should drink Juices to keep well. If there is anything the matter with us, then we certainly should drink Juices, and plenty of them, every day. What Juices to drink? Why? How can Juices be made, to extract ALL the Vitamins and Mineral elements contained in vegetables and fruits? This book points out in a masterly and convincing manner WHICH Juices to use—and why.

This is the only book we have ever found that contains authoritative information on vegetable juices and JUICE THERAPY based on more than 25 years of research and first hand experience.

Thousands upon thousands of copies of this book have been bought the world over—because people want dependable and authoritative information on vegetable juices.

This book describes 150 ailments so the layman can understand their cause and origin, and do something about them. Juices and their combinations are indicated which have given consistently beneficial results. Learn how to combine your juices, and in what proportions.

INDEX

Fresh Vegetables And Fruit Juices

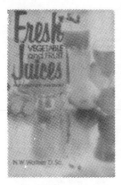

In FRESH VEGETABLES AND FRUIT JUICES, R. D. Pope, M.D., writes—"Dr. Walker has, for the first time in history, written a complete guide of the Therapeutic uses of our more common, every-day vegetables when taken in the form of fresh, raw juices. It will be of considerable help to those who wish to derive the utmost benefit from the natural foods which God created for the nourishment of Man." Dr. Walker categorically lists vegetable juices, explains their elements, and in cooperation with Doctor Pope, provides suggestions for effective treatment of special ailments.

Colon Health: The Key To A Vibrant Life

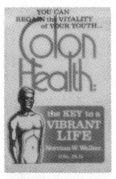

In COLON HEALTH Dr. Walker will take this forgotten part of your body and focus your full attention on it—and you'll never again take it for granted! This books shows how every organ, gland and cell in the body is affected by the condition of the large intestine—the colon. COLON HEALTH answers such questions as: Are cathartics and laxatives dangerous? Can colon care prevent heart attack?—Is your eyesight affected by the condition of your colon?—What are the ghastly results of a colostomy?

Vegetarian Guide To Diet And Salad

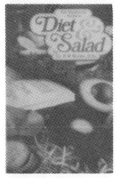

The pitfalls of overindulgence in certain food elements, especially oil and sugar, have been well documented. Dr. Walker offers in his book DIET & SALAD both a cook book and a nutritional guide that belongs in every homemaker's kitchen. In it he supports current medical research about the harmful effects of milk—"It is generally assumed that cow's milk is one of our most perfect foods... Milk is the most mucus forming food in the human dietary, and it is the most insidious cause of colds, flu, bronchial troubles, asthma, hay fever, pneumonia, and sinus trouble... cow's milk was never intended for a human infant."

Water Can Undermine Your Health

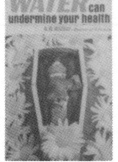

Dr. Walker sees water pollution as a cause of arthritis, varicose veins, cancer, and even heart attacks—a major problem in virtually every community in the country. His treatment of water pollution is revealing, comprehensive, and scientific. His findings, and his recommendations for corrective action, offer new hope.

Educational Wall Charts

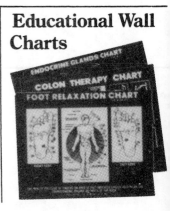

Become Younger

BECOME YOUNGER might be called the "cornerstone" of the famous Walker Program. What place has nutrition in the scheme of good health? How can the body and mind be so tuned that "old age" might be defeated? Dr. Walker suggests 'When we embark on this program which may change our eating, drinking and living habits, we must have the courage of our convictions based on the knowledge which we can acquire through the principles involved in this program... To "become younger" means to have attained a state of sublime *self-reliance* and *self-sufficiency which no one can take away from us."*

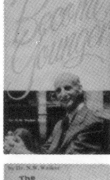

The Natural Way To Vibrant Health

PROPER NUTRITION IS TANTAMOUNT TO GOOD HEALTH. One man today is walking proof of all this. Dr. NORMAN W. WALKER, a living example of VIBRANT HEALTH, has had the answer since 1910. His information is timeless. The originator of "juice therapy," he made this statement in the preface to one of his books: "The lack or deficiency of certain elements, such as vital organic minerals and salts, and consequently of vitamins, from our customary diet is the primary cause of nearly every sickness and disease." For three quarters of a century MEDICAL EVIDENCE HAS NOT REFUTED HIM.

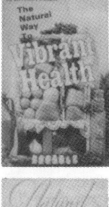

Natural Weight Control

In NATURAL WEIGHT CONTROL, Dr. Walker offers "A Diet Like No Other"– based on the body's need for vital, life-giving enzymes found only in nature's pure foods. On enzymes he writes– "Enzymes are not things or substances! They are the life-principle in the atoms and molecules of every living cell. The enzymes in the cells of the human body are exactly like those in vegetation, and the atoms in the human body each have a corresponding affinity for like atoms in vegetation."

Easy Weight Control with NEW FOOD COMBINING PLAN

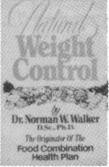

ENDOCRINE GLAND - See where they are located - their innumerable functions, what elements compose them, what Juices nourish them.

COLON THERAPY - A most complete chart of the human Colon. It indicates the relation of nerve endings from head to foot registered in the Colon, and should alert you to study your own condition and to something about it.

FOOT RELAXATION - The soles of your Feed can help relax tension in various parts of your body. This chart shows the Zones on the Soles of the Feet in relationship to the rest of your body.

7" x 22" — IN COLOR

Back To The Land For Self-Preservation

In BACK TO THE LAND Dr. Walker examines urban life. His years of working for better health and nutrition have enabled him to see that now is the time to really come to grips with this dilemma.
He offers inspirational thoughts on living your life with a purpose, and "Enjoying the Life-Style of Your Dreams."

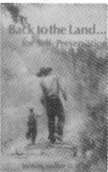

INFORMATION REQUEST & ORDER FORM

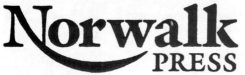

107 NORTH CORTEZ
SUITE 200
PRESCOTT, AZ 86301

Date _____

NAME _____

STREET ADDRESS _____

CITY _____

STATE _____ ZIP _____

QTY.	TITLE	PRICE	TOTAL
	Diet and Salad - Vegetarian Guide to	$5.95	
	Fresh Vegetables and Fruit Juices	$5.95	
	Vibrant Health - the Natural Way to	$5.95	
	Water Can Undermine Your Health	$4.95	
	Become Younger	$5.95	
	Back To The Land for Self-Preservation	$4.95	
	Colon Health: The Key To A Vibrant Life	$5.95	
	Weight Control, Pure and Simple	$5.95	
	Endocrine Chart	$5.00	
	Foot Relaxation Chart	$5.00	
	Colon Therapy Chart	$5.00	

— POSTAGE CHART —
☐ 4th Class Mail - Add $1.25 Per Item
☐ 1st Class / U.P.S. - Add $1.75 Per Item

Sub-Total $ _____

_____ Items X $ _____ Per Item $ _____

Enclosed is my: ☐ Check ☐ Money Order **TOTAL AMOUNT** $ _____

ALL ORDERS SHIPPED SAME DAY AS RECEIVED
- FOREIGN ORDERS: U.S. FUNDS - MONEY ORDER -

FREE INFORMATION

On services and items suggested or mentioned in Dr. Walker books, please check items you are interested in:*

IN-HOME
☐ **DETOXIFICATION Program**

HOME
☐ **VEGETABLE JUICERS**

HOME
☐ **FOOD DEHYDRATORS**

HOME
☐ **COLONIC EQUIPMENT**

☐ **WATER DISTILLERS**

Dr. Walker has no financial interest in any service or product mentioned in his books.

Year after year Modern Medical Science continues to prove...Dr. Walker is right.

INFORMATION REQUEST & ORDER FORM

Norwalk PRESS

107 NORTH CORTEZ
SUITE 200
PRESCOTT, AZ 86301

Date _____

| NAME | _____ |

STREET ADDRESS _____

CITY _____

STATE _____ ZIP _____

QTY.	TITLE	PRICE	TOTAL
	Diet and Salad - Vegetarian Guide to	$5.95	
	Fresh Vegetables and Fruit Juices	$5.95	
	Vibrant Health - the Natural Way to	$5.95	
	Water Can Undermine Your Health	$4.95	
	Become Younger	$5.95	
	Back To The Land for Self-Preservation	$4.95	
	Colon Health: The Key To A Vibrant Life	$5.95	
	Weight Control, Pure and Simple	$5.95	
	Endocrine Chart	$5.00	
	Foot Relaxation Chart	$5.00	
	Colon Therapy Chart	$5.00	

– POSTAGE CHART –
☐ 4th Class Mail - Add $1.25 Per Item
☐ 1st Class / U.P.S. - Add $1.75 Per Item

Sub-Total $ _____

_____ Items X $_____ Per Item $ _____

Enclosed is my: ☐ Check ☐ Money Order **TOTAL AMOUNT** $ _____

ALL ORDERS SHIPPED SAME DAY AS RECEIVED
- FOREIGN ORDERS: U.S. FUNDS - MONEY ORDER -

FREE INFORMATION

On services and items suggested or mentioned in Dr. Walker books,
please check items you are interested in:*

IN-HOME
☐ **DETOXIFICATION Program**

HOME
☐ **VEGETABLE JUICERS**

HOME
☐ **FOOD DEHYDRATORS**

HOME
☐ **COLONIC EQUIPMENT**

☐ **WATER DISTILLERS**

Dr. Walker has no financial interest in any service or product mentioned in his books.

Year after year Modern Medical Science continues to prove...Dr. Walker is right.